THE NEW SE

STOMACH ULCERS AND ACIDITY

Explains the causes of these common complaints
and shows how to avoid and treat them.

THE NEW SELF HELP SERIES

STOMACH ULCERS AND ACIDITY

PRACTICAL MEASURES TO HELP YOU AVOID AND TREAT THESE PAINFUL STOMACH DISORDERS

LEONARD MERVYN
B.Sc., Ph.D., C.Chem., F.R.S.C.

Thorsons
An Imprint of HarperCollinsPublishers

Thorsons
An Imprint of HarperCollins*Publishers*
77–85 Fulham Palace Road,
Hammersmith, London W6 8JB.

First published in *The Science of Life* series
This edition published 1990
3 5 7 9 10 8 6 4

© Thorsons Publishing Group 1990

Leonard Mervyn asserts the moral right to
be identified as the author of this work

A catalogue record for this book
is available from the British Library

ISBN 0 7225 2257 6

Printed in Great Britain by
HarperCollinsManufacturing Glasgow

Contents

Note to Reader

Foreword

Stomach and duodenal ulcers occur as a culmination of rejecting Nature's warnings over a period of years. Ulcers in either the stomach or duodenum don't just happen, they are often the result of years of wrong eating habits, worry or stress, or failure to cope with our modern lifestyle and ignorance concerning how our body functions and how we can best look after it.

Man was never intended to live in our huge 'civilized' cities in an environment which is foreign to his 'natural' habitat. For centuries, in our Western civilization, man lived in a rural or semi-rural atmosphere. Even the big cities of 100 years ago were small in comparison to the sprawling metropolises we know today. During the past fifty or sixty years life has become much more complex, complicated and hazardous as we continue to make what we choose to call 'rapid progress'. No longer do we obtain fresh milk direct from the dairy, but in bottles or cartons which may be a few days old or, if it has been subjected to ultra high temperature processing, it may be several months old. We eat more processed, ready prepared and take-away foods. In Australia one leading dietitian has said that 'one third of all meals are prepared or eaten away from the home and the public don't know what they are getting'. On top of this government statistics show that 25 per cent of all kilojoules (calories) available to the Australian public come from alcohol or sugar. It is little wonder then that we see an ever increasing incidence of stomach and digestive disorders. Our food is not what it used to be and consequently we have paid the price of deteriorating health.

Not all progress is bad, however, and if we can adjust our way of living and our way of thinking to accommodate change we can do much to reap the benefits offered by our modern civilization without losing our health or the quality of life we have been accustomed to enjoy.

Stomach ulcers are usually carefully nurtured and grown with loving care by the sufferer who is usually totally ignorant of what he is doing. Before an ulcer develops there are usually warning signs, digestive upsets and minor discomfort for months and very often for years before the ulcer becomes apparent. It is by paying attention to Mother Nature's warning signs and by successfully overcoming minor digestive problems that more serious disorders including gastric and duodenal ulcers can be avoided.

The digestive tract can be broadly divided into four sections. There are the mouth and oesophagus (gullet), the stomach, the duodenum and small intestine and the colon or large bowel. The chemistry of these four sections varies alternately from alkaline to acid. The mouth and oesophagus are alkaline, the stomach is acid, the duodenum and small intestine are alkaline and the colon or large bowel is acid. It is imperative that each section maintains its normal alkalinity or acidity for normal digestion and that each stage of digestion be satisfactorily completed before the food passes to the next section for further processing.

Digestion begins in the mouth and if food is not chewed thoroughly and completely mixed with saliva before passing to the stomach, digestion in the stomach is impaired. Anyone who suffers with any digestive problem should chew their food for at least twice as long as they are accustomed to do. Remember that you cannot overchew your food. Eat at a leisurely pace and chew it well.

Food transit time through the digestive system is also important. The food only remains in the mouth for a few minutes. In the stomach it takes from 2½ to 5 hours before the food is ready to pass to the duodenum. It takes a further 3½ to 4½ hours for the food to pass through the duodenum and small intestine before it reaches the large bowel. It should then pass through the large bowel in another 12 to 15 hours making a total transit time of about 20 hours. In our Western diet with its predominance of refined carbohydrates, alcohol, sugar and fat transit time can be as long as 72 hours! This means that many toxins from waste products can be reabsorbed into the system giving rise to all manner of illnesses. It is also important to realize that over 90 per cent of nourishment from our food is absorbed from the first half of the small intestine, some 3 to 5 hours after we have eaten it. Little absorption occurs after the food has proceeded past this point.

Food transit time is influenced largely by the type of food we eat and also by exercise. Physical exercise is essential to normal digestion and it is usually sedentary workers who suffer with digestive problems although manual workers are not immune from them, particularly if they eat their food quickly, wash it down with tea or coffee and visit the local pub regularly after work. To maintain normal food transit time adequate fibre must be included in the diet, so too must a plentiful supply of fluids, preferably water. It is unwise to drink with meals. Most people who drink with meals do so because they fail to chew their food thoroughly and so have to wash it down instead of mixing it with saliva and enabling it to slip down the gullet easily. Drink twenty minutes after a meal, not while eating.

Our Western diet also contains an excess of fat, sugar and salt. These should be reduced but not excluded from the diet. Stimulants such as tea, coffee and alcohol should be avoided.

What happens once an ulcer has developed? How do we overcome it and prevent it from recurring? That is just what this book is all about. There are many simple, easy-to-follow measures which can be employed to assist ulcer sufferers. Correct diet, simple herbal remedies, overcoming stress and learning to live in our present day environment are all important to the ulcer sufferer. The value of foods such as yogurt, herbs like slippery elm bark and liquorice, vitamins and minerals are all explained simply and clearly. If you do not have an ulcer this book will show you how to avoid it; if you are unfortunate enough to suffer with one then this book contains much valuable information to help you overcome it.

1

The Digestive System

Before we consider and discuss the various aspects of gastric and duodenal ulcers it is important to understand the whole process of food digestion. Not only is food subjected to a superbly controlled sequence of processing from the time it enters the mouth to its eventual excretion; at each stage digestive juices of the right type and make-up play their part in reducing the food to a form in which it can be absorbed and utilized by the body. We need a digestive system because food constituents as presented in the diet are complex substances that have to be reduced to simpler ones before the body can assimilate them. Basically, during the process, starches and sugar are digested or hydrolysed to the simplest sugar glucose. Proteins are reduced to their individual amino acids, some twenty or so in all. Fats and oils are emulsified then broken down to their constituent fatty acids and glycerol, which are partially re-combined after absorption to produce the type of fats that the body needs. Some of the glucose remains to be used as fuel for the workings of the body but most of it is built up into animal starch called glycogen which forms part of the fuel reserves, ready to be split once more into glucose when required.

The amino acids derived from the food are absorbed as such then combined by body processes to produce the proteins specifically for the human body. Some amino acids are set aside for other uses, for example, as brain and nerve transmitters; others can be utilized as fuel and inter-converted to make other amino acids. Fats represent a very important energy reserve since they are readily broken down and fed into the energy-producing cycle, like glucose, but they do have other specific functions. These are usually well catered for so that the problem is usually too much rather than too little fat laid down as energy storage depots.

It is relatively easy to break down the basic food constituents in the laboratory or in a factory. Boiling starches and proteins with acid will produce glucose and amino acids respectively. Boiling fats and oils with alkali will yield the free fatty acids (as sodium salts) and glycerol as in making soap. The digestive process is much less drastic although the end results are the same.

The body utilizes enzymes that are specific protein (organic) accelerators or catalysts that under certain conditions will break down the food constituents just like acids and alkalis do but in a more gentle manner. These enzymes require other constituents and narrow limits of acidity and alkalinity to digest food efficiently and the digestive processes are geared to supply these. Of course, digestive enzymes despite being proteins in structure, are not affected by the conditions under which they act in the digestive tract but are usually de-activated as they move through with the food at the next stage.

We shall now look at the process of digestion as it occurs at the various levels of the gastro-intestinal tract. The first stage happens in the mouth but even before food is introduced into it, various stimuli have caused the digestive juices to be produced. Even whilst the meal is being prepared, the smell of the cooking food, the thought of the taste to come and the anticipation of satisfying the appetite causes the saliva to flow. At the same time gastric juices, very potent in acids and enzymes, are secreted. Lower down in the twenty-two feet of small intestine other juices are being produced in readiness for the anticipated food. Apart from salivation the most obvious sign of the approaching meal is the gurgling of the stomach juices although this can be a symptom of hunger even without food in the offing!

The Mouth

The saliva produced by specific salivary glands in the mouth is there to lubricate the food and assist in the actions of chewing, cleaning the mouth and swallowing. In addition it contains an enzyme, ptyalin, that converts starches into maltose, a sugar that is almost at the ultimate stage of digestion. There is some doubt regarding the signifi-cance of this early digestive process since starch is readily digested further down the system. The efficiency of ptyalin depends upon how long the food is chewed; in animals that bolt their food, salivary ptyalin is absent.

The functions of the mouth and tongue are thus essentially to prepare the food for the main digestive processes further down the tract. They assist in the mastication of food and its formation into a bolus; they assist in swallowing. In addition the tongue is the sensory organ for the appreciation of taste, texture and temperature of food. Taste and texture are the stimuli to keep the digestive fluids flowing after their initial response to the smell of food.

These senses too are the first line of defence against eating food that is 'off'. The nose is the first to spot it and the usual reflex action is to spit out the obnoxious food. If some has already been swallowed both taste and smell will exert their protective actions by telling the stomach to refuse to pass the food on. The reverse process comes into play so the bad food is squirted back into the mouth from where it is readily vomited. The whole process is usually preceded by nausea so there is plenty of warning that the food is about to be rejected. Sometimes the food may have been passed on through the stomach to the intestine. This is usually the point of no return since there is a valve preventing intestinal contents from going back into the stomach. In such an instance the intestinal muscles will react by passing the poisonous contents quickly through the rest of the digestive tract. The end result is diarrhoea that disposes of the noxious material, eliminating it from the body. Hence although unpleasant, nausea, vomiting and diarrhoea are essentially protective and beneficial mechanisms.

The Oesophagus or Gullet

Although the oesophagus does not contribute to
the digestive process, it links the mouth and the
stomach. The walls of this connecting tube push
the food into the stomach by a process of peristalsis
which is simply alternating contraction and relaxation of the muscle. Gravity also contributes but
peristalsis is the main process since thanks to this it
is perfectly feasible to swallow when standing on
one's head. There is some sort of valve, albeit not a
very efficient one, between the oesophagus and the
stomach so there is a little slowing down and
control of the passage of food into the stomach.
Usually however, the food passes fairly quickly
into the stomach after swallowing. We shall see
later how reverse movement of stomach contents
into the oesophagus gives rise to a distressing
condition called oesophagitis.

The Stomach

The stomach and the rest of the alimentary tract
are shown in their relationships in Figure 1.
As the food is chewed the fluids produced by the
salivary glands and the stomach continue to flow.
The food is pulped with the teeth, tongue and the
insides of the cheeks and mixed thoroughly with
saliva. Eventually it is neatly packaged together at
the back of the tongue where there are specific
nerves that are stimulated to induce the act of
swallowing. Once anything touches these nerves
swallowing becomes an involuntary reflex action
and nothing can stop the food or drink from
entering the oesophagus.

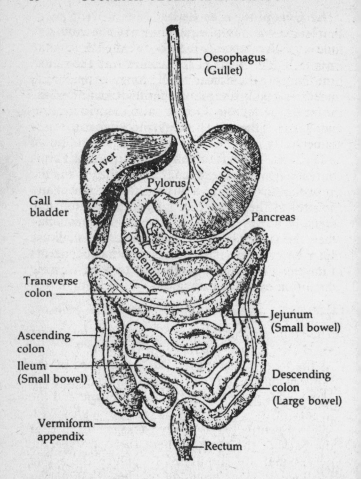

Figure 1. The digestive system

Note the length of the duodenum, the long, narrow neck which connects the stomach to the small intestine. About 75 per cent of ulcers occur in the duodenum.

Adjacent to the oesophagus is another entrance that leads down to the lungs or up into the nose. As food is swallowed a small soft body called the uvula rises to block off the nasal passages; at the same time the larynx (leading to the lung) is sheltered under the epiglottis so preventing food from entering the lungs. Food is thus directed down the oesophagus and as we have seen, it inevitably enters the stomach.

The stomach is of variable shape according to its contents and has the capacity to expand. It lies in the upper abdominal cavity, more to the right than the left. It is here that the digestive process really starts. Its action is like that of a washing machine where the pulped food gets turned over and over so that the various digestive juices can reach all parts of it. The walls of the stomach are rich in glands which secrete many substances. They include:

(a) Mucin, a protein that acts to protect the walls of the stomach from acid.

(b) Gastric juice which contains pepsinogen, which is inactive itself but is converted to the enzyme pepsin by another secretion, hydrochloric acid. Pepsin starts the breakdown of proteins. Another component, rennin, curdles liquid milk protein called caseinogen into the solid protein casein. This is then acted upon by pepsin.

(c) Hydrochloric acid which creates an acid environment essential for the digestive enzymes to work. At the same time this acid can disinfect the food destroying harmful bacteria. It also destroys ptyalin the salivary enzyme. Hydrochloric acid also controls the pylorus which is the valve that functions between the stomach and the next length of small intestine known as the duodenum.

(d) Hormones called gastrins are also secreted and they have the function of keeping up the flow of gastric juice until the meal is digested. Gastrins also stimulate the release of intrinsic factor from the stomach walls and as we shall see later, this factor is absolutely essential for the absorption of vitamin B_{12}.

(e) Lipases which help digest fats are also secreted in the stomach but their significance is doubtful since fat digestion is mainly the province of the intestine.

The stomach has a unique function not only as a processing chamber but also as a food store, for it has the capacity to expand to hold large quantities of food at a time. Drink that enters the stomach with food is passed on very quickly but some is mixed with the food, softening it further. Then it is squirted, a little at a time, into the next part of the gastro-intestinal tract, the duodenum. At this stage the stomach contents are known as chyme.

The Duodenum
The duodenum is about twelve inches long and is like a horseshoe in shape. It comprises the first part of the small intestine. It leaves the pylorus valve at the stomach and encircles the head of the pancreas to which it is firmly attached. It lies mainly to the right of the midriff and continuous to the next bit of the intestine called the jejunum.

The duodenum receives juices from two sources, the pancreas and the liver, via the pancreatic duct and bile duct respectively. Both juices are strongly alkaline so that in addition to their other functions they serve to neutralize the highly acidic chyme being squirted in from the stomach. The alkaline conditions that result in the duodenum act as the ideal medium in which the enzymes secreted in the duodenum can continue with the digestive process.

Pancreatic fluid is not only efficient in liquefying the partly digested proteins and the starches present in the food from the stomach but it has also the capacity to attack the fats in it. Bile assists in this because it contains bile salts, such as sodium glycocholate and sodium taurocholate, that emulsify fats and oils, rather like washing-up detergents that remove fatty residues from dirty plates.

The enzymes present in pancreatic secretion are:

(a) Trypsinogen, inactive until converted to the active enzyme trypsin. This digests proteins and partly-hydrolysed proteins almost to amino acids.

(b) Chymotrypsinogen, inactive until converted to the active enzyme chymotrypsin by the other enzyme trypsin.

(c) Amylase, a starch-splitting enzyme that converts both starch and glycogen (animal starch) almost to glucose.

(d) Lipase, a fat-splitting enzyme that causes hydrolysis of fat to fatty acids and glycerol. This enzyme is activated by bile salts which are produced in the liver and secreted in the bile.

(e) Carboxypeptidase, secreted as inactive pro-carboxypeptidase but produced by the action of the other enzyme pepsin. The end result of carboxypeptidase digestion is some amino acids and combined amino acids called peptides.

The Small Intestine

The duodenum takes up only the first twelve inches of the small intestine. The rest is made up of the jejunum which is eight feet long and the ileum which comprises the last twelve feet.

Digestion is completed by enzymes secreted in the intestinal juices which are produced by the glands of Brunner and of Lieberkuhn. These enzymes are:

(a) Aminopeptidase and dipeptidase which between them complete the digestion of proteins to simple amino acids.
(b) Disaccharidases which complete the digestion of the products of digestion by amylases (pancreatic enzymes) to glucose.
(c) Lipases that are specific for digesting complex fats like lecithin.

The small intestine, along its whole length, is also the main site for absorption of all the products of digestion which are now in a suitable state to be absorbed.

Hence the small intestine performs both digestive and absorption functions. It is often abused yet continues in its efficient manner. When we consider the hot spices; the unnatural cooked food; the over-cooked or even burnt food items; the pips, stones, bits of paper, coins, even fragments of broken glass that we present the gastro-intestinal tract with, it is a miracle that the small intestine continues to digest and absorb. It can be polluted with medicines, alcoholic drinks, drugs, and infective micro-organisms yet it still carries on.

In spite of these abuses the stomach and the small intestine and indeed the rest of the intestinal tract continue to work virtually twenty-four hours a day, churning up food, kneading it, mixing it with self-made juices, squirting it for hours on end until almost every constituent of the food has been reduced to its basics. These basics are glucose, amino acids, fatty acids, vitamins and minerals. The only constituent not reduced further is dietary fibre but even this has an important function, as we shall see later.

Absorption of these basic food constituents is an intricate process and the cells of the lining of the small intestine are particularly adapted for it. They comprise a highly specialized absorbing surface which is so finely and intricately folded that the total surface area is about that of two tennis courts! This is necessary because of the sheer volume of the food and digestive fluids passing down the small intestine. Every day we make almost three gallons of these fluids in order to digest our food and most of this volume has to be absorbed back into the body or we would die of dehydration. This is why we can continue to suffer from diarrhoea even after drinking nothing – in this case all the fluids are not absorbed. Persistent diarrhoea can be dangerous, particularly in babies and small children, because they are unable to replace the huge losses of water being excreted. This is why fluids are often introduced directly into the vein, to bypass the diseased gastro-intestinal system.

The stomach does not absorb anything apart from alcohol. This explains why the euphoric effect of alcoholic beverages is so rapid – absorption starts as soon as the stomach is reached. The ill-effects of alcohol appear much later because the body takes time to start disposing of the substance and it is the first metabolites like acetaldehyde that are toxic.

The Large Intestine
The large intestine, which is about six feet long, starts with the caecum which joins the end of the ileum at the ileocaecal valve. After this comes the ascending colon which bends at a right angle to continue as the transverse colon then turns through another right angle downwards to form the descending colon. The end of the colon (also called the large bowel) is the pelvic colon which joins to the rectum. This is the end of the line as far as food residues are concerned because the rectum ends in the anus, the excretory exit for the faeces.

The ileocaecal valve allows the food residues from the small intestine to go through into the caecum a little at a time. By this time the residues have less and less digestible material left with proportionately more of the indigestible plant fibre – cellulose and lignin – derived from fruit, vegetables and bran. In addition there is a very large quantity of bacteria present. These bacteria are the so-called 'friendly' ones that are beneficial to us, helping in the rotting-down process of the vegetable constituents in the food we eat. During this process they produce some B vitamins and the fat-soluble vitamin K. A proportion of these are absorbed so that we can make use of them and they contribute to our daily allowance of certain vitamins.

Strong antibiotics unfortunately kill these good bacteria, as well as the harmful ones, sometimes to such an extent that our intake of B vitamins and vitamin K is seriously reduced. For this reason these vitamins are sometimes prescribed with antibiotics. If they are not, it is still useful for an individual to take a vitamin B complex product whilst on antibiotics and for a short period afterwards. Destruction of 'friendly' bacteria can also cause diarrhoea so freeze-dried preparations of them in powder form or even living yogurt can help by supplying fresh colonies.

The food has been digested and its nutritious components absorbed by the time it reaches the beginning of the large intestine. It is still however semi-fluid and the function of the large intestine is to extract most of the remaining water. This conservation of water in our body is important since if it were allowed simply to go through the rest of the system, dehydration would soon result. The mass of food residue plus bacteria is steadily pushed along the large intestine, losing more and more water along the way, and finally ending up as a solid mass. In this form it is stored near the end of the large intestine where accumulation takes place before the final excretion.

This mixture is now faeces and at a certain time, usually after breakfast, it is transferred *en masse* into the rectum. The rectum responds by telling the brain that it wants to rid itself of this material and the end-result is the desire to defecate or 'open the bowels'. Under normal conditions this is complete. The semi-solid faeces are extruded in the characteristic sausage form which in fact reflects the shape of the lining of the rectum. The act of defecation to completion immediately produces a strange feeling of well-being and satisfaction. At the same time it must be remembered that this material is not normally poisonous or harmful. It consists mainly of undigested fibre and harmless bacteria that can continue this 'rotting-down' process even after leaving the body. The brown colour of normal faeces is derived from bile pigments – the smell comes from the decomposition process caused by the 'friendly' bacteria.

Although most of the food constituents of our diet are digested then absorbed, the undigested fibre plays an important role throughout the digestive tract. Because they cannot be digested, fibres such as these found in bran, fruit and vegetables survive throughout the whole system and add bulk to the food contents. This bulk enables the whole of the gastro-intestinal system to carry out its peristaltic action in moving the food, even when mainly digested, along the tract. At the same time, these fibres absorb water and in so doing they swell, giving the walls of the gut a solid mass to work on. At the excretory end fibre is really important since its bulk and water-retaining capacity enable the faeces to maintain a semi-solid state. Constipation is due to over-absorption of water resulting in hard, compacted faeces; diarrhoea is the retention of too much water by the faecal mass. Hence dietary fibre can help by normalizing the water content of the excreta in both cases.

It seems that even soluble, indigestible food fibres like guar gum and other vegetable gums have an important part to play in the absorption and excretory systems. When dissolved in water, these gums act like a gel which also supplies bulk to the food mass. As gels they perform two very important functions. They slow down the absorption of sugars, so preventing a massive rise in blood sugar occuring after a meal. In addition they retain water and hence present bulk to the faecal constituents, aiding the insoluble fibres in their functions.

2

Indigestion and Related Conditions

There are many conditions associated with the stomach and adjacent parts of the digestive tract that can be a prelude to or consequence of gastric ulceration and excess acidity. These can be prevented or treated by sensible eating and care in the diet. Knowledge and correct diagnosis of these conditions and their early detection and treatment can often prevent the occurrence of the more serious peptic ulceration and its consequences.

Simple Indigestion

Eating too much denatured and processed food, eating too quickly, and eating badly prepared or ill-assorted combinations of food, can all bring on an attack of acute indigestion. This is also known as dyspepsia but no matter what it is called, it causes much discomfort. Sometimes this is relieved by vomiting which is Nature's way of curing it. More often though there is a very unpleasant feeling of nausea. Relief can be gained by drinking heavily salted water or, more drastically, by sticking two fingers down the throat. These heroic measures are not often needed however. Relief is often obtained simply enough by getting some cool, fresh air on the face or having a drink of cold water. Many people will experience a bloated, distended feeling often amounting to pain. One common cause is the result of air swallowed during the meal but it may also be due to nervousness. A meal that has lasted too long is often the reason. The best relief, embarrassing as it may be, is often a good belch. An attack of hiccups, though perhaps just as embarrassing, is usually the end-result.

For these symptoms there are many traditional remedies that are helpful – amongst the most pleasantly effective are the liqueurs taken at the end of a banquet. Originally this was why they were produced and drunk traditionally at the end of a meal and all are based on natural aromatic oils. Orange, peppermint, aniseed and dill are amongst the most popular and effective plant oils. Such oils are known as carminatives and in the hands of the herbalist are used extensively in the relief of flatulence. No one is quite sure how these oils in liqueurs settle the stomach but the alcohol content plays no part. Relief from flatulence is just as easily obtained from peppermints, orange slices, root ginger or essential oils from these plants. Just as important as taking this treatment is the half-hour rest after a heavy meal. In babies, gripe-water has the same carminative effect and it is worth remembering that this remedy can be just as effective in adults.

These treatments are all natural ones; to attempt to deal with the condition by taking strong medicine or alkaline powder is not the way to clear up the trouble. The price of purchasing a little momentary relief by these means is to render yourself more and more open to future attacks. Such treatment merely treats the effect. It makes no attempt to remove the cause which lies largely in our traditional feeding habits.

Both rich meals and alcoholic drinks have a dehydrating effect, probably because, as we have seen, vast amounts of digestive juices are needed to cope with the food and the body will draw on its reserves of water to supply them. Alcohol, by virtue of its properties, will literally draw water out of the body tissues. The simplest remedy to ensure against suffering the day after over-indulging in food and drink is to drink not less than a pint of water before going to bed. This makes up the balance of the water previously lost and is the best natural treatment. As we shall see, however, it is simpler and better not to over-indulge but look more closely at what you eat and drink.

Occasional indigestion, particularly in the evening, can often be relieved by other natural means. Try getting extra sleep by going to bed early or getting up late. Take at least two hours exercise in the open by walking, golfing or gardening. Eat only light portions of food such as fish and fresh fruit. Carry on drinking large volumes of non-alcoholic drinks like natural, unsweetened fruit juices to keep down the calories but increase your vitamin C intake. In all circumstances avoid sleeping pills. Don't be misled by taking 'the hair of the dog' alcoholic drinks. This is a complete fallacy as it is now known that alcohol can only delay recovery. Give your digestive system a chance to recover – don't overload it with the very foods that caused the trouble in the first place.

There are always people who seem to develop indigestion easily and frequently, almost to the extent of daily discomfort. Often such attacks occur after consuming rich red wines, spices or citrus fruits. Although frequent attacks may give the individual the impression that there is something medically wrong, this is not often the case. It is a nuisance that can be prevented by sensible eating. It is often quite erroneously assumed by such individuals that they are allergic to these and other food items. Real food allergies are quite different and often result in copious vomiting, diarrhoea and skin reactions that give rise to blotchy, itchy rashes and patches. True allergy can make the unfortunate individual very ill indeed. Once allergies have been professionally identified, the only remedy is to avoid the food items causing them. Simple indigestion is only very rarely due to an allergy.

Nervous Indigestion

The simple indigestion discussed above can have a variety of causes including, as we have seen, allergies to food constituents. In addition to these physical causes however we must also add those due to psychological trauma. In this case nervous tension is often the culprit; a condition that can be brought on by stress, worry, external pressures or even an imminent examination, interview or some other event. Too often the immediate treatment is to take sedatives and tranquillizers to calm the nerves since these are the basis of the problem. This approach is most unwise since these drugs only create much worse problems of drug dependence, depression and drowsiness which in turn dulls the mind. Look instead to the cause of the nerviness. Self-examination may often be sufficient to rectify it. If you feel the need of a calming-down agent, seek a herbal preparation or a high potency vitamin B complex formulation. These are mild, safe, non-habit forming and function through natural methods on the nervous mechanisms.

When we consider that we do not consciously tell our digestive system to work it is obvious that to a large extent the nervous control of the whole digestive process is not under our own control. Nevertheless since nervous indigestion is a fact of life conscious thought can stimulate the flow of juices, perhaps when we don't need them, and contractions of the stomach and the rest of the digestive system. The nerves that tell our system these things reside in a large, multi-functional nerve called the vagus. This supplies many other organs of the body as well as the digestive tract so it is not surprising that mental factors can affect the workings of the stomach. In fact, one treatment for over-production of stomach acid and chronic indigestion is by cutting the vagal nerves that supply the stomach but this drastic therapy is now often replaced by less invasive treatments.

Chronic Indigestion

Many attacks of indigestion are temporary and giving the stomach a rest is often all that is needed for relief. Some people, however, do appear to suffer a constant discomfort after eating. This may be related to habitual wrong feeding and is aggravated rather than helped by the taking of one or more of the patent medicines on the market. Treatment therefore resides in a change in diet and it is gratifying to see how often this does the trick. This approach is dealt with later in the book but if, despite sensible eating, chronic indigestion persists it is sensible then to seek professional medical advice.

Heartburn

This is due to the acid stomach secretions regurgitating into the gullet, giving a burning sensation. This reflux of the stomach contents often happens when one is lying down after a heavy meal or even by bending down. Such heartburn is not unusual since it is simply related to the position of the body but if it happens in the upright position it means that the contractions of the stomach are actually pushing the acidic contents up into the gullet. They have managed to force their way through the ring of muscle between the gullet and stomach which, although not quite a sphincter or valve, usually manages to contract to hold the juices back. Although the stomach has an internal surface able to cope with acid, the oesophagus does not and it reacts by causing pain and burning sensation. The pain is known as heartburn and it is quite descriptive since it is frighteningly similar to the pain of some heart attacks. Again, if it happens only occasionally it may pass or it can be treated with a natural oil like peppermint but if it occurs consistently it should be treated by other means. It can be the cause of a disease called oesophagitis (see page 35).

People who are overweight have a greater tendency to suffer from heartburn. It can also happen in those with a malformation at the lower end of the gullet so that some of the stomach lies in the chest. This is called a hiatus hernia (see page 38).

'Indigestion' due to Wind

Whenever food, liquid or simply saliva is swallowed air usually accompanies it. This is just ordinary air that happens to be in the mouth at the time of swallowing. There is vast individual variation in the amounts of air swallowed; some people swallow several gallons during the course of a day. Even new-born babies swallow air. At birth there is no air in their stomachs but it is introduced as soon as they are able to swallow. Suckling is notorious for introducing air into a baby's digestive system resulting often in pain and discomfort that can only be relieved by a burp.

Usually we do not notice swallowed air but you can guarantee that it is always there. Only when it reaches large volumes does it become uncomfortable producing a relieving belch. The problem is that we invariably swallow more air in preparing to belch, only to bring it up again.

Too often, it is possible to get into the habit of associating the occasional ordinary feeling of mild discomfort in the stomach with 'a little bit of wind'. Attempts to belch it up cause more air to be swallowed, more discomfort and the whole cycle to start again. The end result is a glorious belch that was totally unnecessary in the first place as air was introduced as a deliberate action. Ignore ordinary, occasional mild twinges in the abdomen and don't exacerbate the condition by introducing unnecessary air.

It is amazing how often it is believed that 'wind' forms in the stomach. It does not. All air within the gastro-intestinal system has been swallowed. One of the most common abdominal complaints in the world is that of 'wind' but it is not a disease and singly reflects the bad habit of swallowing air. Belching may be considered a compliment to the chef in some parts of the world but it never justifies a visit to a practitioner nor does it indicate a dietary or digestive disorder.

Oesophagitis
Oesophagitis (inflammation of the oesophagus or gullet), gastritis and peptic ulcers are responsible for the vast majority of indigestion pains and difficulty in swallowing. We shall therefore consider each in turn but diagnosis of each particular complaint must be left to the practitioner.

The oesophagus is ostensibly a very simple structure but its mobility is similar to that of the gastro-intestinal system. At the top end it has a sphincter (or valve) that acts as a barrier to accidental swallowing because it is usually constricted, except when swallowing. The lower sphincter, connecting with the stomach, is less well defined but it is a barrier sufficient to prevent continual reflux (bubbling up) of gastric contents into the bottom end of the oesophagus. It is more of a kink than a developed valve but combined with a slightly higher pressure in the oesophagus it usually prevents regurgitation of stomach contents.

The lining of the oesophagus simply provides mucus to lubricate swallowing, rather like saliva does in the mouth. Although the lining of the lower end may secrete a tougher mucus to stand up to acid gastric contents it is not able to withstand them for long and the burning pain of oesophagitis is due to a direct action of this acid on the lining of the oesophagus.

The oesophagus is a relatively simple structure and there are only a limited number of mechanisms operating in its disorders. The most usual are physical obstruction, an inefficient valve, direct damage and bleeding. Obstruction may be caused by a foreign body; a growth; muscular uncoordination of the valve; a spasm or by a stricture or narrowing of the tube due to scar tissue from a previous injury. Sometimes the valve fails to relax or open and when this happens the main symptom is difficulty in swallowing.

An inefficient valve will allow the gastric contents to squirt up into the oesophagus, causing inflammation and pain. Damage to the oesophagus can be caused by swallowing any corrosive substance or, in some cases, medicinal drugs. The antibiotics tetracyclines, the anti-spasmodic drug emepronium bromide, and the mineral supplement ferrous sulphate are the main offenders but there are other drugs that can cause a similar inflammation if incompletely swallowed. Bleeding in the oesophagus can be due to a variety of causes but the most likely is scarring of the lining with sharp foods like crisps, crushed boiled sweets and the like. Oesophagitis is made worse by smoking and drinking alcohol. Coffee and popular drugs like aspirin can also exacerbate the condition.

Signs and Symptoms of Oesophagitis: The two predominant symptoms of oesophageal disorders are difficulty in swallowing and pain. The cause of the pain is usually mucosal inflammation and is usually described by the sufferer as indigestion or heartburn. The pain is usually located behind the breastbone but it can radiate into the arms or neck. It is usually associated with meals or with certain foods; with posture, being intensified by bending forwards or lying back, and with the sensation of regurgitation, perhaps even into the mouth. These signs and symptoms are characterisitic of the condition 'reflux oesophagitis'.

If the pain is due to oesophageal spasm it is much less characteristic and more easily confused with the pain of a heart condition. It is, however, relatively rare. Loss of appetite and possibly nausea may also result from pain in the oesophagus, no matter what is the cause.

Bleeding from the oesophagus is very rare. However, any vomiting of blood is serious and requires medical attention. Unchanged blood, red in colour, suggests the origin of the bleeding is the oesophagus. On the other hand, partly digested blood that is colourfully described as 'coffee grounds' suggests it has arisen in the stomach or duodenum.

Difficulty in Swallowing (Dysphagia)

We have all experienced 'a lump in the throat' for emotional or other reasons and it makes swallowing difficult, uncomfortable or even painful. Anxiety and depression can cause the same sort of feeling and is often the reason for the 'relaxed throats' that are common in tense or nervous people. If the oesophagus is blocked or paralysed by disease however, it is possible to swallow quite easily but instead of carrying on down, the food stops moving and may be regurgitated into the mouth. Although sometimes secondary to pain, this type of difficulty in swallowing may be due to more sinister causes and professional help should be sought.

Hiatus Hernia

Hiatus hernia is a distinct anatomical defect where the sphincter between oesophagus and stomach is displaced from its normal site at the point level with the diaphragm where the oesophagus joins the stomach (see Figure 2). There are two types of hiatus hernia, the sliding type and the para-oesophageal type. These are also illustrated in the diagram.

In the sliding type of hernia, the top end of the stomach has slid up into the chest. The oesophagus empties into it perfectly well since the sphincter is well into the chest. Food goes down inside the gullet, past the diaphragm muscle and on into the intestine perfectly easily. The only discomfort in some people is that there is easy regurgitation of food back into the gullet from the stomach. The result is an acid heartburn pain just behind the breastbone after meals.

This sort of hernia is a minor problem and treatment of it is easy. If it is due to overweight, the painful regurgitation will stop once the individual loses weight. The reason is that once this happens the pressure inside the abdomen will no longer tend

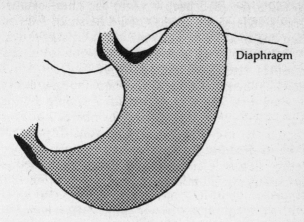

A para-oesophageal hernia

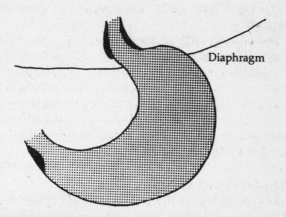

A sliding hiatus hernia

Figure 2. Types of hernia

to force the food back up into the chest against gravity. Hence all meals should be small ones so that the food will go down easily and stay down. Another tip is to stay sitting upright for a few minutes after each meal so that the food stays down. When these relatively simple measures are carried out, the discomfort of a sliding hiatus hernia will cease. It must be remembered however that if the individual is of a nervous disposition they may continue to suffer from simple nervous indigestion as described above. Sliding hiatus hernia is usually symptomless and hardly ever requires a surgical operation. It has been calculated that some 30 per cent of the population suffer from it. Sensible eating habits are still the best and easiest way to control the condition.

On the other hand, para-oesophageal hiatus hernia is more likely to give symptoms and requires rather more attention. The reason that this type of hernia is more serious is that the part of the stomach that lies in the chest is so placed that it cannot slide freely up and down. It may get trapped and hence suffer serious damage. Determination of which type of hiatus hernia is present requires professional diagnosis but either condition can be relieved by simple diet.

Acute Gastritis
Acute gastritis is really inflammation of the lining of the stomach. Its other name is acute erosive gastritis. It is usually caused by ingestion of alcohol, aspirin or other drugs, food and drug allergies or toxins from staphylococcal food poisoning. Some-

times the condition accompanies such apparently unconnected diseases like those of the kidney and infections like influenza. Other causes include, over-eating, the unwise combination of foods, or one or more of the dietetic indiscretions listed in this book. Usually gastritis is the stomach's definite indication that it can no longer tolerate the foolish and indiscriminate manner in which it has been fed and treated. It then proceeds to stage a strike against all further food until the whole digestive tract has been cleaned out – which is a somewhat painful and exhausting procedure.

Symptoms of acute gastritis are commonly lacking but loss of appetite, nausea, vomiting and gastric pain after eating may be present. Very occasionally the stomach lining may actually bleed. Treatment is usually aimed at withdrawing the offending agent, whether it is a medicinal drug or an allergic food. Changing the diet or ceasing to take alcoholic drinks will also relieve the condition. Fortunately the lining of the stomach regenerates itself very rapidly. Once the cause has been identified and removed, the self-healing process takes over and the stomach returns to normal after one or two days.

Corrosive Gastritis

This complaint is usually caused by swallowing strong acids, strong alkalis, concentrated iodine, potassium permanganate solutions or heavy metal salts like lead, mercury and cadmium. Gastric damage varies depending upon the nature and amount of the ingested poison. Often ulceration of

the lips, tongue, mouth and throat will give a clue
to the cause of the condition. Dysphagia or difficulty
in swallowing suggests the oesophagus has also
been damaged. The main symptom is severe abdominal pain sometimes accompanied by gastric bleeding.

The antidote and treatment depend upon the
specific agent and amount taken and on the time
interval before treatment. Acids are neutralized by
alkalis and vice versa so here the antidote is fairly
obvious. Other poisons may need expert advice,
however, since induction of vomiting which may
appear obvious may simply transfer the poison
from the stomach to the gullet, throat and mouth
where its corrosive action continues.

Chronic Gastritis

This is where the lining of the stomach is persistently
inflamed but no one is quite sure what the cause is.
Recent evidence suggests that the passing back or
reflux of bile into the stomach is to blame. The bile
acids have been particularly implicated in the
condition since these are known to cause erosion of
the stomach lining. Chronic gastritis is often a
feature of gastric ulceration and in some cases may
be the cause. Hence the dietary suggestions to
prevent and treat gastric ulcers that are discussed
later (page 118) should also help in overcoming
chronic gastritis. Apart from dietary treatment
there is no other effective therapy for this distressing
condition.

Dyspepsia

Dyspepsia is a condition in which the nerves of the

stomach inhibit normal digestion and cause stomach acidity. Flatulence and gas pains are common. The typical dyspeptic is a neurasthenic. That is to say, his digestive troubles arise out of his restless, unrelaxed nature. He eats without discrimination at irregular intervals, leads a restless, ill-planned life, and subsists on a diet sadly deficient in all natural nerve foods and vitamins. He often smokes too much, drinks a lot of coffee, tea or spirits and fails to obtain sufficient sleep.

3

Peptic Ulcers, Their Symptoms and Causes

The number of people who suffer chronically from stomach or duodenal ulcers, acidity, dyspepsia or indigestion is appalling. No statistics are available, but unofficial estimates by medical men are to the effect that one person in every three over the age of thirty is either a chronic or partial sufferer from some kind of indigestion, gastric upset, or ulceration of the digestive tract. The pain and misery of these people as the result of their meals cannot be computed in terms of unhappiness.

It has been estimated that some twelve per cent of the adult population of Australia suffer from a stomach ulcer or its forerunner, chronic indigestion, after every meal. In Britain, medical authorities have estimated the number of sufferers from these two stomach ailments to be in the vicinity of four million. In the USA some authorities claim that as many as ten million people or more suffer from peptic or duodenal ulcers or acute, chronic indigestion. No club, no bar, no place where people meet is complete without its group of ulcer sufferers, and the doubtful humour which accompanies them. But ulcers are no joke. They are tenth among the list of chronic diseases as a cause of death and twelfth as a cause of absenteeism. American experts reckon that one out of every ten people is now bound to have a peptic ulcer sometime before they die.

Gastric ulcers occur mostly in early life. Duodenal ulcers usually pester middle age. Most ulcers are small – from a quarter of an inch to an inch in diameter. But they have an unpleasant habit of boring inwards through the walls of the stomach or duodenum rather than spreading along the surface. That's why ulcers kill. If they perforate those walls, you may die. Before we proceed, let us define the various types of ulcers to which human beings are vulnerable.

There are four times as many cases of stomach and duodenal ulcers among men than women, and for reasons which we will discuss later. The typical 'ulcer type' is generally lean, energetic, and anxious. Fat, placid men rarely get stomach ulcers. This is not to suggest that the lean, energetic type of person need get them – that to this type, stomach ulcers are inevitable. There is absolutely no need for any human being to become a victim of this painful – and highly dangerous – form of suffering that makes life a misery. Indeed, the suffering is incalculable, and the tragedy of it is that it is all so unnecessary. The consistent application of a few sensible principles can not only cure it, but can restore health to the highest level and keep it there.

What is a Peptic Ulcer?
Any ulcer is defined as an open, concave lesion of

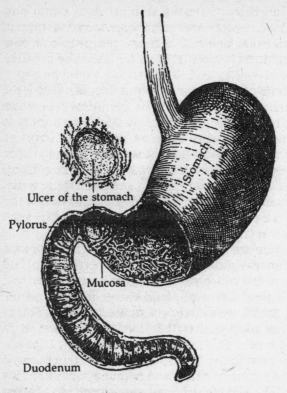

Figure 3. A stomach ulcer
An ulcer of the stomach, shown in the usual location, just at the pylorus, or exit of the stomach. The duodenum is shown below the stomach, and connects it with the small intestine.

The stomach of the average human adult secretes about three quarts of gastric juices daily. Gastric juices contain hydrochloric acid, pepsin and rennin. These digest food by chemical reaction.

varying depth in the skin or mucous membrane. In the case of peptic ulcers, they are erosions through the mucous membrane that lines the gastro-intestinal tract, penetrating the muscular layer and even the blood capillary bed. Although we associate peptic ulcers with the action of stomach acid eroding the membranes, the digestive or 'peptic' enzymes also contribute. Hence the term peptic ulcer applies to those found in the stomach itself (gastric ulcer); the first few inches of the duodenum (duodenal ulcer); the lower end of the oesophagus (oesophageal ulcer), and that formed at the sphincter between stomach and duodenum, called a pyloric ulcer.

All types of peptic ulcer are the result of acid and peptic enzymes. The acid is hydrochloric, a strong acid that is needed for digestion, for sterilizing food that may be infected or water that is contaminated. It is thus an essential secretion in our stomachs – later we shall see the serious consequences of the conditions where no acid is produced, known as achlorhydria. More likely, however, is the over-production of hydrochloric acid and hence the over-production of the peptic or digestive enzyme. What happens is that acid and enzymes leak back into the oesophagus causing ulceration. In the stomach, the most likely area for erosion by acid and enzymes is that of the lesser curvature of that organ. The most common form of ulcer however is found in the first inch or so of duodenum where the acid gastric contents first contact the duodenum lining. This lining is less resistant to acid than that of the stomach and erosion can take place before the alkaline secretions of the duodenum can effectively neutralize the acid gastric contents.

Peptic damage can vary widely in its effect. In its mildest form it may be present merely as inflammation, the best example of which is alcohol-induced gastritis. There may be small erosions most likely associated with certain drugs like aspirin and the anti-inflammatory medicines used in treating arthritis. The most severe form is a single large cavity that can reach half an inch in diameter, which is the classical peptic ulcer.

Since the gastro-intestinal tract has an inherent self-repair process, an ulcer is in a continuous state of flux with phases of damage and repair attending with each other. Examination by endoscopy (see page 52) hence reveals an inflamed active ulcer, full of exudate. In the quiescent repair stage that same ulcer appears as pale pink scar tissue.

The current view of peptic ulcer is that it is the result of an imbalance between normal erosive processes going on constantly and the ability of the tissue of the gastro-intestinal system to protect itself. Too much acid and digestive enzymes shifts the balance to the erosion side. In addition to these, however, must be included irritant drugs such as aspirin, anti-arthritic drugs, corticosteroids, iron salts, alcohol and bile. All of these can damage the lining of the stomach and duodenum.

What then are the protective factors? First and foremost is a thin layer of alkaline mucus secreted by the stomach lining. Production of this protective layer depends upon a healthy mucous membrane with the ability to have a fast turnover of cells to replace the inevitable losses. Replacement of these cells which produce the mucus, in turn depends upon various factors such as a good blood supply and protective hormones called prostaglandins. Both factors are the result of a good diet with an adequate supply of both vitamins and minerals so our food can play a big part in protecting us against peptic ulcers.

What are the Symptoms of an Ulcer?

The symptoms caused by ulcers are basically pain, the discomfort often making the sufferer belch as a result of trying to 'bring up the wind'. The pain is often quite characteristic in the way it comes and goes. Remember though that most instances of stomach pain have nothing to do with ulcers at all. These conditions were discussed in Chapter 2.

We have seen that the stomach can develop other disorders apart from ulcers even though the symptoms may be similar. The most common symptoms are loss of appetite, nausea, retching, vomiting and loss of weight. Even these can be due to emotional problems; disgust, for example, can easily cause nausea and vomiting; painful stomach cramps can arise from simple anxiety.

The usual symptoms of stomach ulcers are intense pain, vomiting, and occasional haemorrhage. The pain is the most consistent symptom, and may come on from half an hour to two hours after eating. Those with duodenal ulcers experience exactly the same symptoms, only in their case pain is felt a little to the right of, and above the navel, instead of in the stomach itself. There is usually a longer time lag between the meal and the pain.

Here are some of the many easily recognized symptoms of ulcer:

- Chronic indigestion.
- Acid stomach.
- Acid belchings.
- Gas.
- Heartburn.
- Gassy distention.
- Burning sensation in the stomach.

In more severe cases these symptoms are present:

- Indigestion that appears about two hours after eating.
- Indigestion and stomach distress that suddenly stops when more food is eaten.
- Pain in the stomach.
- A sore spot in the stomach that is tender to pressure.
- Vomiting.
- Haemorrhage.
- Black-coloured stools. (They are black because of stomach haemorrhage.)
- Yellowing of the skin. (Caused by absorption of blood substance mixed in the food from bleeding ulcers.)
- Anaemia from loss of blood.

Of course, all of the symptoms may not be seen in every case of stomach ulcer but any one is a very suspicious indication that an ulcer is at work. Pain after meals is the most common and most certain symptom.

New York Specialist on Ulcer Symptoms

Dr Joseph F. Montague, a noted New York specialist, wrote the following useful outline of the symptoms of stomach ulcer and duodenal ulcer:

> Stomach or duodenal ulcer starts a warning signal swinging in nine cases out of ten. That warning is pain, and the ulcer patient gets it invariably at some time of the day or night, if not at both of these periods, in the form of a sharp feeling of distress or a gnawing sense of discomfort. Whatever form the pain manifests itself in, it is well to heed it, for with ulcers generally an ounce of the good old prevention is worth the traditional pound of cure.
>
> Very often when symptoms of so-called indigestion appear, the patient doses himself with this or that nostrum, or contents himself with taking a nightly purge. In the minds of many men there persists the belief that a physic will cure practically every ailment of the human body. So, the stomach ulcer patient, conscious of a burning sense of distress in his stomach, beneath his breast bone or between his shoulder blades, takes this or that laxative in the naive belief that he can wash his trouble out of him. Such purgatives are a positive menace where an ulcer is present, for they irritate tissue and stimulate peristalsis to a point that causes bleeding.
>
> Duodenal ulcer, on the other hand, often has little effect upon the patient's weight. His appetite remains fairly normal and his only awareness of trouble in his digestive tract is the distress that comes along after he has eaten, or when he is about to eat again.

How Ulcers are Located

To find out if you have an ulcer, a doctor will

probably test the contents of your stomach before and after eating, and X-ray your stomach before and after you have eaten barium, which has a metallic content and therefore shows up on an X-ray photograph. If you have a chronic, deep ulcer the barium, an opaque substance, will fill up the hole the ulcer has left and reveal it. But it won't show up all ulcers, so your doctor may be left guessing whether that queer mark on your X-ray plate means that you have an ulcer or that you just have some kind of irritation.

With the increase of ulcer cases, medical science has devised a clever way of looking into the stomach. This is called cystoscopy. Scientists have produced a flexible tube with a system of lenses and electric lights and tiny mirrors which can be swallowed quite easily. It allows the operator to see inside the stomach, and even to take coloured photographs. A normal stomach has thick, smooth, orange-red folds. An ulcer looks like a small volcanic crater set in a red plush curtain!

Incidentally, most ulcers – three out of four – occur in the duodenum. The duodenum is the narrow neck of the stomach which connects it with the small intestine. Also, ulcers are more frequent among men than women, due chiefly to the fact that during their middle years, their stomach acid reaches a higher level. They eat more rapidly than women, and are likely to wash their meal down with tea, coffee, or beer, which are all acid-forming.

The Differences Between Duodenal and Gastric Ulcers

The causes of both types of ulcer are fundamentally different. Lack of the mucosal protection is the prime cause of gastric ulcers. When combined with irritation and inflammation of the stomach lining induced by various factors, a resulting ulcer is almost inevitable. The lack of a good blood supply to an area of the gastric mucous membrane also probably plays a part.

Duodenal ulcers are more likely to be a result of overexcretion of acid and peptic enzymes. The contact time between the duodenal lining and the erosive contents of the stomach as they pass into the duodenum also determines the susceptibility to duodenal ulcers. This can be prolonged for a variety of reasons and the chances of ulceration are increased. The effect of chronic stress is associated more with the developement of duodenal than with gastric ulcers. Acute stress is more likely to cause gastric ulcers.

The pain of duodenal ulcers is often relieved by food; that of the gastric type is aggravated. Night pain is more a feature of duodenal ulcers. The development of cancer can be a feature of gastric ulcers but there is no association between it and duodenal ulcers.

Risk Factors for Peptic Ulcers

Stress remains one of the most important factors for the development of so-called 'acute stress ulcers'. The term embraces not merely psychological stress but also the metabolic stresses associated with severe illness, burns, surgery, and accidental injury, all of which can produce peptic ulceration as a secondary feature. Other factors include smoking, group O blood, drugs, and a family history of gastric or duodenal ulcers. Although stress and medicinal drugs, because of their irritant action, may seem to be understandable factors, we are still uncertain as to why men are three times more prone than women to develop peptic ulcers. Nor do we understand why duodenal ulcers are three times as common as the gastric type. The fact that some five per cent of gastric ulcers become cancerous whilst duodenal ulcers rarely do is another mystery.

What are the Causes of Peptic Ulcers?

There are many causes, and most victims have for many years been guilty of not one, but several of the following:

- Over-eating
- Worry.
- The use of aluminium cooking utensils.
- Too much starchy food.
- Incompatible food combinations.
- Vitamin and mineral deficiencies.
- Mixed, messy and indiscriminate feeding.
- Hasty eating and improper mastication.
- Condiments
- Sugar consumption.
- The laxative habit.
- Alkaline powders.
- Weakened resistance of the blood to noxious bacteria.

These causes are not necessarily listed in order of importance, and generally a combination of several of them is responsible for the ulcer. Let us examine them in some detail:

1. Over-eating: Most people eat more food than they need for energy and the repair and maintenance of bone and tissue. All excess food puts an added strain on the digestive mechanism. Often it breaks down under the strain, and digestive troubles result.

2. Worry: The brain and the stomach are connected by the vagus nerve. Tests have shown that when a person is worried the flow of the powerful gastric juices in the stomach is increased. Indeed, under such conditions it continues to flow, whether food is present in the stomach or not. If there is the slightest ulceration in the stomach, the constant flow of the gastric juices – which contain hydrochloric acid – irritates the ulceration and enlarges it. On this point, Dr Richard Harrison has written:

> The stomachs of people with severe nerve weakness are in a constant state of irritation and unrest.
> This is because the nerves that stimulate normal stomach activity do not stop working when the stomach is empty.
> Instead, a continuous flow of irritating stomach juices is produced. On the walls of an empty stomach this continual, unnatural flow of stomach juices has a damaging effect.
> The stomach, after all, is a piece of meat. And stomach juices are designed to digest meat (and other protein foods).

Under ordinary conditions, Nature furnished good
protection for the stomach tissues against its own
juices. But when stomach tissues are continually
saturated with a wholly abnormal amount of digestive
fluid, some area loses the ability to further protect
itself from damage . . . An ulcer or ulcers is the result.

The destructive emotions of anger, rage, hate,
jealousy and fear all have disastrous effects upon
digestive processes. Meals eaten under mental or
emotional tension lead to inadequate mastication,
giving rise to faulty digestion. Worry and anxiety
interfere with normal digestive activity.

3. The Use of Aluminium Cooking Utensils:
Aluminium is a soft metal, readily affected when
used for cooking foods because it is soluble in both
acids and alkalis. Most foods have either an alkaline
or acid reaction.

Traces of oxide of aluminium, when combined
with sodium chloride (common salt) from the
cooking of vegetables in salt water, and ingested
with food, adversely affect the health-giving potassium in the human body. There is also evidence
that these tiny particles of aluminium enter the
stomach and weaken the stomach lining with their
astringent properties, thus encouraging the formation of ulcers.

4. Too much starchy (and protein) food: Processed
and refined starchy foods – bread, flaked, puffed
and toasted cereals, porridge meals, cakes, pies,
biscuits, rice, macaroni, etc. – constitute the bulk of
the diet of the vast majority of the population. Both

processed, starchy foods and proteins are acid-
forming and an excess of these foods in the diet
upsets the proper acid-alkaline balance and leads to
acidity – the forerunner of all digestive troubles
(and, incidentally, of rheumatism and arthritis).

Alkali-forming foods, which are more desirable,
include vegetables, fruits and most nuts, apart
from Brazils and peanuts. Remember, however,
that foods are acid- or alkali-forming only after
absorption and assimilation by the body. Whilst in
the digestive system, fruits, for example, contribute
citric, malic and other acids. Although these are
weak compared with the strong hydrochloric acid
that the body produces itself, they do contribute
some acidity.

The important point about food and the diet in
general is to ensure that each meal is balanced.
Food constituents themselves, particularly the
proteins, have a neutralizing or buffering action on
stomach acids that can help prevent the effects of
over-production. There is no such action by starches
and sugars.

5. *Incompatible food combinations:* Although a
balanced meal, in respect of its various food constituents, is considered to be highly desirable by
some authorities for the prevention of digestive
problems this is not agreed by everyone. There is a
modern school of medical thought which attributes
much of the digestive troubles of men and women
to the common practice of eating protein and
starch foods, or acid and starch foods, at the same
meal.

The starches referred to are – bread, packeted cereals, porridge meal, pastries, biscuits, jams, ice-cream, etc. These starch foods do not combine well in the stomach with protein foods (meat, fish, eggs and cheese) or with acid fruits (oranges, grapefruit, tomatoes, pineapples, peaches, plums, apples, apricots, etc.). This kind of 'incompatible feeding' often leads to gas, fermentation, flatulence, pain, and finally to chronic indigestion, dyspepsia, and/or ulceration.

The most sensible advice, however, is to be 'middle of the road' when it comes to eating meals, i.e. moderation in all things without excessive intake of any one particular food item, no matter how good you may think it is.

6. *Vitamin and Mineral Deficiencies:* It is no exaggeration to say that 90 per cent of the entire population suffers from vitamin and mineral deficiency of some sort. If this were not so, there would not be over 3,000,000 admissions to public and private hospitals every year in Australia, for example, and people would be far healthier.

In the case of digestive and ulcer sufferers, there is abundant evidence that these unfortunate people have long been deficient in vitamins A, B complex, C and E, and in calcium.

Vitamin A is required for the health of the epithelial tissue (i.e. the inside of the mouth, the tonsils, trachea, lungs, intestines, lymphatic glands, and the walls of the stomach, pylorus and duodenum). This vitamin has been shown in medical trials to be effective in accelerating the healing of peptic ulcers (see page 86).

The B complex vitamins are essential to the health of the nervous organization and the secretion of enzymes necessary for good digestion.

Vitamin C is required for healing any ulcer. Vitamin C builds healthy connective tissue and strengthens the walls of blood vessels. It also helps to stimulate 'antibodies' and phagocytes which destroy bacteria in the blood-stream.

Vitamin E acts most beneficially upon the heart and muscles. It dilates the capillaries and permits an improved flow of blood to congested areas. It also dissolves blood clots. Lack of this vitamin in the ordinary diet appears to have some bearing upon the increase in the number of stomach ulcers.

Calcium is important to the health of the body. Without it, the nerves and muscles cannot relax, giving rise to tension. Without Vitamin D (which we mostly obtain from sunshine) and phosphorus, the body cannot utilize the calcium in our food supply.

7. *Mixed, and indiscriminate feeding:* Most of us have grown up in the evil dietetic tradition that all so-called food is good for us – that it's all 'grist for the mill'. We therefore proceed to eat anything and everything that comes our way, regardless of the appalling task we have set our digestive organs, our eliminatory organs, and the chemistry of the body itself. Soup, meat, vegetables, puddings, washed down by tea or coffee – down it all goes! We may feel satisfied after such a meal but we have set in motion the ingredients which finally create fermentation, flatulence, acidity, hyperacidity, and stomach

trouble. If that were not bad enough, our next meal may add to the offence by consisting of one or other of the doubtful concoctions found in the delicatessen shop. Here we see a picturesque assortment of embalmed, preserved and demineralized products, masquerading as 'food' in the form of pies, pastries, pickled pork, pickled onions, corned beef, pigs' trotters, and an assortment of sausagemeats, consisting of meat scraps, flour, fat, colouring, and artificial flavouring and seasoning. All these products are alleged to feed you, but in reality they will hasten the onset of the pains of stomach ulcers and ill health.

A generation less notorious for its educated ignorance would condemn all such foods as unfit for human consumption. Very hot drinks, highly spiced foods and ice-cold drinks and foods all irritate the stomach lining. Sufferers from stomach troubles should also abstain from alcohol which increases the acidity of the stomach.

8. *Hasty Eating and Improper Mastication:* Every one must surely realize the digestive troubles they are inviting by eating meals under mental tension, leading to improper mastication and digestion. It is recognized by medical science that worry, anxiety and stress interfere with the normal activity of the stomach and that anger, rage and fear tend to over-excite and over-activate the flow of gastric juices.

9. *Condiments:* A further potent cause of ulceration is the habit of taking condiments. We have come to depend upon the artificial stimuli of mustard, pickles,

pepper, chutney, tomato sauce, salt, etc., to give us an appetite. But all these products are harmful irritants. They certainly stimulate appetite by exciting the flow of gastric juices but it is unnatural stimulation. The result is to leave the appetite more jaded than ever, so more stimulants are used, and so on. The result is that the lining of the stomach is subjected to such irritation that it becomes inflamed and finally ulcerated.

10. *Sugar Consumption:* Sugar, whether white or brown is a refined, concentrated carbohydrate completely divorced from all the beneficial elements of the original sugar cane. It is sweetness without sustenance, devoid of the essential vitamins and minerals. Molasses, the residue of sugar cane, has nutritional virtues. But sugar is left with only the dangerous delusion – the highly refined crystals that please the eye, seduce the palate and increase acidity. But in spite of its pleasant appearance and taste, sugar is a slow, insidious poison, robbing the body of its calcium by neutralizing it, setting up fermentation and acidity, and slowly but remorselessly undermining the health of its host. If you value your health, don't use sugar. If you want a substitute, use honey, which contains both vitamins and minerals.

At one time, it was usual to over-emphasize the factors of stress and strain as the dominant cause of stomach ulcers. However, research done in the 1960s showed that there are fewer ulcers among top-ranking businessmen than among lower paid people doing routine jobs. The survey found that shift workers in particular are very prone to ulcers.

It also revealed that there are more stomach ulcers among townspeople than country dwellers, not because there is more stress in town living, but because townspeople eat more sugar. Moreover, stomach ulcers are now not uncommon among children, doubtless due to an unbalanced diet containing a high proportion of sugary foods, refined cereals, soft drinks, sweets, ice-cream, chewing gum, etc. More attention than ever before is now being directed to faulty nutrition as the real cause of stomach ulcers.

11. *The Laxative Habit:* The taking of laxative pills and medicines is a notorious contribution to ulceration and inflammation of the digestive tract, especially the stomach. These laxatives are irritants; foreign bodies, which cause fermentation and unnatural stimulation of the nerves, muscles and mucous membrane of the stomach and alimentary tract. One authority explains their internal reaction as follows:

> When a purgative of any kind is introduced into the system, its presence is a constant irritation to the sensitive mucous lining of the bowel. The intestines react against the purgative, and in forcing it out of the system a bowel action necessarily takes place. But mark the fact that the action is brought about by the expulsion of the salts, or whatever it is, which the body regards as something foreign and repugnant to it.

It is now known that the regular use of laxatives can give rise to serious, even incurable, intestinal ailments in later years. Proper feeding will bring about regular bowel movements without pills or purgatives and the evils they lead to in the digestive system.

12. *Alkaline Powders:* Sufferers from digestive troubles or stomach ulcers usually seek refuge in one of the antacid powders or bicarbonate of soda preparations on the market. They feel that because these alkali powders give some relief from the pain and flatulence which follow every meal, they must be counteracting the acidity and so assisting in the healing of the ulceration. This is not the case, however. The antacid powder or bicarbonate of soda habit will in time make the condition worse. It does nothing to remove the cause of the trouble.

Dr William Howard Hay was once asked if antacid powder or bicarbonate of soda should ever be used to relieve indigestion or 'sour stomach' and he replied:

Not if used to correct stomach acidity, for it would aggravate the very thing for which relief was intended. Sour stomach comes from either an over-supply of hydrochloric acid or from the various fermentations of the carbohydrate foods (starches and sugars).

If from too much of the stomach acid mentioned, then correction by the soda merely means that enough or more of this acid will be secreted to continue the interrupted protein digestion, thus increasing the habit of formation of this, while if due to fermentation, this merely neutralizes the acids without in any way stopping the fermentation, which proceeds at the old rate.

The B complex vitamins, vitamin C, calcium, and iron, all need an acid medium in the stomach in which to carry out their various functions in promoting bodily health. Bicarbonate of soda, antacid powders and other alkalizers produce an artificially alkaline condition in the stomach, thereby neutralizing the action of the vitamins and minerals which are lost to the body.

13. *Weakened Resistance of the Blood to Noxious Bacteria:* This is the logical outcome of nutritional deficiencies and defects in the mode of life, so usual with the digestive and ulcer sufferer.

4

THE ROLE OF
HYDROCHLORIC ACID

If you look up a chemistry text-book you will see
hydrochloric acid described as a colourless fuming
aqueous solution of hydrogen chloride gas with a
very pungent odour. Yet this same acid in a dilute
form is an important part of the human digestive
system and its excess or lack can have profound
effects upon the health of the individual. When too
much is produced the condition is known as hyper-
acidity and this is one of the factors contributing to
the formation of peptic ulcers. When too little is
formed, the condition is called hypoacidity and the
net result can be less effective digestion in the
stomach. In some cases no acid at all is produced
and the condition is referred to as achlorhydria.
The absence of hydrochloric acid will increase the
chances of developing gastric cancers.

Before we consider these various aspects of
hydrochloric acid production, let us see how it is
made within the stomach.

The Production of Hydrochloric Acid
In the lining of the stomach there are two types of
secretory glands. One consists of a single layer of

secreting cells known as chief cells which produce digestive enzymes. The other type of secretory gland consists of cells arranged in layers. They are known as parietal cells which secrete hydrochloric acid directly into the gastric glands and hence into the stomach. The mixed secretion is known as gastric juice. It is normally a clear, pale yellow fluid of high acidity, (between 0.2 and 0.5 per cent hydrochloric acid) but with 97 to 99 per cent water. Also present are the protective protein mucin, inorganic salts and digestive enzymes.

Hydrochloric acid is a combination of hydrogen ions (which determine acidity) and chloride ions. Hydrogen ions arise in the following manner. Carbon dioxide which is present in blood plasma as a normal respiratory component passes into the parietal cell. This cell has blood plasma on one side with the opening of the stomach on the other. Within the cell there is an enzyme, called carbonic anhydrase, which catalyses the reaction between carbon dioxide and water to form a weak acid known as carbonic acid. This is the same acid that is formed in carbonated drinks like lemonade. Because it is weak, carbonic acid readily dissociates into bicarbonate plus hydrogen ions. Bicarbonate cannot leave the parietal cell to enter the stomach but readily passes back the other way into the blood. The second component of hydrochloric acid, chloride, is always present in the blood (this is why blood tastes salty) and readily passes through the parietal cell and into the stomach itself. Here it combines with the hydrogen ions already produced by this specific cell and the net result is free hydrochloric acid.

Bicarbonate is alkaline and, as we have seen, this passes back into the blood. Hence after a heavy meal when hydrochloric acid is produced in great quantities, a lot of bicarbonate is also formed at the same time. This upsets the balance of acids and alkalis in the blood and it is then up to the kidney to restore the balance by getting rid of the extra bicarbonate into the urine. The end-result is the so-called alkaline tide which simply means that the urine is alkaline instead of slightly acid as normal. Alkaline urine promotes bacterial growth so too many 'alkaline tides' can eventually give rise to urinary infections.

Why do we Need Hydrochloric Acid?

This acid, along with some weaker organic acids that are also secreted into the stomach, provides the right sort of acidity that is essential for the first digestive enzymes to work. The digestion of proteins starts under the influence of the enzyme pepsin which cannot function unless the pH (measure of acidity) is between 1 and 2. Hydrochloric acid is essential for the gastric juices to reach this low pH (anything below pH7 is acid and the stronger the acid the lower the pH).

There is another enzyme, also secreted by the stomach, that requires a very acid medium in which to work. This is rennin and its main function is to coagulate milk into a solid form that can be acted on first by pepsin then by other enzymes further along the gastro-intestinal tract. Lack of hydrochloric acid will therefore make milk more difficult to digest.

It must be pointed out however that those people who have had the whole stomach, or just that part that produces acid, removed are still able to digest proteins and milk. Their digestive processes may not be quite as effective as they would be with a normally functioning stomach but it does suggest that the roles of pepsin and rennin are not quite as critical as was once thought.

The presence of hydrochloric acid, however, becomes of prime importance in the liberation of vitamin B_{12} from food and its eventual absorption. In meat, which is the most important provider of B_{12}, the vitamin is attached to proteins and the prior digestion of these proteins is essential for the vitamin to be released. Once it is free, vitamin B_{12} is able to combine with a specific protein called intrinsic factor that is also produced in the parietal cells of the stomach.

This complex of vitamin and intrinsic factor can only be formed in the presence of hydrochloric acid and calcium. Once formed, the complex is then transported intact to the ileum where it is absorbed. If intrinsic factor is not present, vitamin B_{12} cannot be absorbed and the result is the once-fatal disease called pernicious anaemia. Lack of hydrochloric acid will therefore reduce the absorption of vitamin B_{12}. It is not without significance that a major symptom of pernicious anaemia is a complete absence of hydrochloric acid in the stomach.

Increased Secretion of Hydrochloric Acid

We can now look at the factors that can cause an increased secretion of hydrochloric acid and its consequences. Of all the digestive tract, the stomach is one organ which is relatively easy to get at and its response can be studied by observing it in people who by reason of accident or design have a hole in the stomach, known in medical circles as a gastric fistula. The strength and quantity of hydrochloric acid produced by the gastric cells can thus be measured under a variety of conditions.

Psychological moods were found to be amongst the most influential factors in producing excess hydrochloric acid. Anger, worry and anxiety all caused the stomach walls to become red, swollen and inflamed with a marked increase in movement and gross over-secretion of acid. Other studies indicated that similar symptoms became apparent when the person was disgusted, resentful, depressed, fearful or when there was a reason to feel insecure, hopeless or defeated. Significantly, the recall of past frustrations or disappointments alone was sufficient to stimulate excess acid production.

As we have seen, hydrochloric acid secretion is usually the response of the stomach to an anticipated meal. The rumblings and gurgles associated with hunger are the stomach's reactions to the expected influx of food. Once it is eaten, though, the first-secreted hydrochloric acid is neutralized but secretion continues in order to maintain an acid medium.

Certain constituents of food have been found to be more stimulating to acid production than others. High protein foods like meat and fish, and beverages like coffee and tea all have a profound stimulant effect on acid secretion. Bitter materials have been known for years to have a stimulant effect on the appetite; now we know that aperitifs like sherry and campari simply act by causing hydrochloric acid to be produced.

Despite popular belief, highly spiced foods like chilli, curry, pickles, vinegar, soused herrings, mustard and frankfurters have little or no effect upon hydrochloric acid secretion. The burning sensation suffered by some people on taking these foods is more likely due to a localized effect of the 'hot constituents' on the lining of the stomach.

In view of the corrosive action of the highly acidic gastric juice, and the exposure of the stomach mucosa to it, perhaps it is surprising that this lining does not break down more often. If it does, of course, the result is a gastric ulcer. Usually, however, the stomach is able to protect its lining by secreting large quantities of mucus. This mucus forms a tough barrier and confers a high level of protection. It is quite possible that people who suffer from gastric ulcers produce only a thin, weakened type of mucus or possibly none at all.

Even when the ulcer has formed, if a thick layer of mucus covers it, it cannot be attacked by stomach acid and often the gastric lining is then able to heal itself effectively. A traditional remedy for treating gastric ulcers is liquorice and this has been found to act by stimulating the production of a thick layer of mucus over the area of the ulcer. A widely-used drug called carbenoxolone that is succesful in healing ulcers is derived from liquorice.

Other treatments for excessive hydrochloric acid production are simple neutralization with alkalis. Specific drugs and surgery are also used to control the acid production. Surgery involves cutting the nerve, called the vagus, which carries the impulses telling the parietal cells to make acid. Another approach is to use drugs that are known as histamine H_2 receptor antagonists. Since the naturally-produced histamine is a potent stimulator of hydrochloric acid production in the parietal cells, it is logical to use drugs that specifically block the action of histamine upon these cells. Hence acid production is curtailed and in its absence the irritant action is lost and the normal healing processes of the body are allowed to take over and get rid of the ulcer.

We shall see later how too little gastric hydrochloric acid can have serious consequences so it is possible that prolonged reduction in the secretion of acid by surgery or by drugs will increase the chances of these consequences. In a similar manner, constant neutralization of the stomach acid with oral alkalis can have serious effects: first by removing all of the acid so that the desired acidic medium in the stomach is lost; second because neutralization simply stimulates further production of acid so that more alkali must be taken and so on. A vicious circle is set up so that eventually the parietal cells simply give up.

Deficiency of Hydrochloric Acid

A deficiency or complete lack of stomach hydrochloric acid has more far-reaching consequences than an excess. Dietary minerals are solubilized by the acid and this makes them more amenable to absorption. Adelle Davis reported how an orthopaedic specialist found that his patients consistently had low levels of hydrochloric acid. Once the deficiency was overcome by supplementing with the acid, the rate of bone healing and ossification increased as more calcium became absorbed.

She also quoted references supporting the fact that an insufficiency of hydrochloric acid can result from a low intake of protein and deficiency of vitamins A, B_1, B_2, B_6, niacinamide, choline and pantothenic acid. Volunteers deficient in pantothenic acid were found to have reduced hydrochloric acid secretion as well as a decrease in digestive enzymes, other digestive secretions and gastric motility. It required three weeks of high potency treatment with this vitamin before normal secretions and motility were restored. Vitamin C absorption is more efficient in the presence of hydrochloric acid presumably because it keeps ascorbic acid in the free form.

Achlorhydria

A complete lack of stomach hydrochloric acid known as achlorhydria is a feature of several diseases. The most common is chronic gastritis where the parietal cells have been destroyed by atrophy of the gastric mucosa. Cancer of the stomach is usually characterized by achlorhydria, mainly because the tumour envelops the parietal cells so they no longer function. One of the diagnostic features of pernicious anaemia is finding that there is no hydrochloric acid produced. Even when the anaemia responds to vitamin B_{12} injections, there is no effect upon the gastric mucosa and hydrochloric acid secretion is still curtailed. When the stomach is partially or fully removed by surgery, the source of hydrochloric acid disappears so that digestion can only start in the mildly alkaline conditions of the small intestine. In these circumstances and indeed in any other condition where achlorhydria is a feature the consequence is the same. There is an increased chance of cancer in the gastro-intestinal tract. We shall now examine why this is so, and look at the best way to combat it.

One of the more potent group of carcinogens, i.e. cancer producing agents, is the nitrosamines. They are substances known to be associated with increased incidence of cancers of the bladder, the oesophagus and the stomach. Sources of nitrosamines include cigarettes, chewing tobacco and snuff. Even non-smokers are exposed to them by way of sidestream smoke from cigarettes. Betel-nuts contain nitrosamines and as the nuts are chewed, the carcinogens are swallowed and enter the stomach and small intestine. Low levels of nitrosamines are present in cured meat products and malt beverages.

It is not only foods that provide us with nitrosamines. Cosmetics, corrosion inhibitors and a wide variety of rubber products have been found to contain ready-made nitrosamines. Even some rubber teats for baby bottles have been found to be contaminated with these substances.

Nitrosamines can also be formed in the stomach by the interaction of two other food constituents, namely, amines and nitrites. Nitrites are readily formed from nitrates, found, for example, in many vegetables and in drinking water and they are also added to cured meats, bacon, sausages and the like. Nitrites are excellent preservatives which is why they are added to foods.

Amines are natural constituents of foods (for example the characteristic smell of fish is due to them) but are also widely used in cosmetics and drugs. Neither amines nor nitrites are likely to cause cancer on their own but when they react together, the result is the carcinogenic nitrosamines. However, what has emerged from recent research is the fact that nitrosamines are more likely to be formed in a stomach that lacks hydrochloric acid. Once the nitrosamine has been formed it can then act anywhere within the digestive tract or be absorbed and produce its carcinogenic effect elsewhere.

Hence the simplest way to prevent nitrosamine formation is to inactivate the nitrites or the amines. The most effective agents for this are vitamins C and E which harmlessly detoxify nitrites. With these out of the way, there is no chance of nitrosamine formation. At the same time there is evidence appearing that vitamins C and E can also combine with and render harmless the preformed nitrosamines.

It would appear then that an adequate intake of vitamins C and E daily is the best protection against nitrosamimes but it is of even more importance if the stomach has ceased producing hydrochloric acid. For complete effectiveness these vitamins must be taken with food, preferably 100mg of each. If we wish to take hydrochloric acid by mouth what is the best way? It is possible to drink hydrochloric acid in a very diluted form but the practice is not recommended for self-treatment. It is likely to cause damage to the teeth, and heartburn. Usually it is introduced straight into the stomach via a tube so this is a technique reserved for the medical practitioner. There is also doubt as to the efficiency of hydrochloric acid administered in this way. A more useful supplement is to introduce hydrochloric acid in combined, solid form. Betaine hydrochloride is a white powder that can be produced in tablet form. Once dissolved this material yields 25 per cent of its weight as hydrochloric acid. The usual dose is between 60 and 500mg of betaine hydrochloride taken just after meals. Glutamic acid hydrochloride acts in a similar manner but in solution it yields only 20 per cent of its weight as hydrochloric acid. For this reason the recommended intake is 0.6 to 1.8g during meals.

There is no doubt that hydrochloric acid is an important secretory agent of the stomach but like so many other body constituents it is most effective when carefully controlled. Some people will go through life happily unaware of any deviation from the normal state of affairs. For those of the emotional type and who undergo periods of stress there must be an awareness of what excessive hydrochloric acid can do. It is more sensible for them to carry around nuts, dried fruit, protein wafers, malted milk tablets and the like, to counteract any hyper-acidity, rather than alkali tablets. At the other end of the scale, once achlorhydria has been established, hydrochloric acid tablets and, more importantly, vitamins C and E should form part of their everyday supplementation.

5

Orthodox and Natural Treatments Examined

The main causes of acidity, dyspepsia, indigestion and stomach ulcer have already been discussed. People who suffer from these troubles in one of their various forms usually have a medical history which shows that they have long transgressed in more ways than one. Orthodox medical treatment for stomach ulcer usually consists of putting the patient on a 'soft, bland diet', supplemented with medicine. Failing that, surgical operation may be thought necessary.

In the light of advanced medical experience over the last twenty-five years, surgical operations for stomach ulcer are little short of folly, in many cases. Such operations merely attempt to cut off the effect. They make no attempt to remove the cause. Only in the extreme case, where the ulcer has eaten a hole through the stomach wall into the peritoneum, is surgical treatment warranted.

The soft, bland diet generally resorted to in hospitals is suppressive rather than curative. A soft, bland diet usually consists of milk and 'pappy' food. The ulcer is soothed rather than healed. No attempt is made to tell the patient where his diet was at fault. This is borne out by the fact that medical men generally fall victims to the usual catalogue of human ailments just like the people who, in desperation, go to them for advice! Often their diet is no different from that of the general run of the public.

After leaving hospital, ulcer sufferers, for want of better knowledge, invariably resume the very diet that caused the trouble, and generally suffer from the same trouble periodically throughout their lives, often ending in some incurable disease.

The Orthodox Theory of Causation

The orthodox concept does not admit that stomach ulcers are caused by a combination of faults in feeding. We have seen that the most likely cause of ulcers is an imbalance between the ulcer-producing factors like excess hydrochloric acid and digestive enzymes and the protective factors like mucus production, permeability of the lining and the rate at which cells of the lining are replaced. What causes this imbalance?

At one time it was thought that a 'focal infection' was the cause. This theory completely overlooked the fact that a focal infection itself (an abscessed tooth or tonsils) is merely a symptom of deep-seated ill-health and which, in turn, is most probably due to faulty nutrition.

The probability is that infection (from teeth, tonsils, or bowel) or defective blood-supply produces a local area of necrosis – the ulcer – and that the hydrochloric acid, which is always excessive in ulcer, keeps it open.

That was Dr Sippy's theory of ulcer-formation.

In the famous Sippy treatment, therefore, great dependence is put upon the use of alkalis such as bicarbonate of soda and milk of magnesia by mouth, in order to neutralize the excessive acid secretion.

The symptoms of ulcer in the stomach and duodenum are very characteristic. Dr Berkeley Moynihan used to emphasize this by saying that the patient in telling his story seems to be trying to recite the symptoms of ulcer as he remembers them from having read them in a text-book on medicine.

Pain, or, rather, a sense of discomfort or rawness, referred to the pit of the stomach, coming on in the case of the stomach ulcer right after meals, in the case of the duodenal ulcer when the stomach is empty or just before meals, is the main symptom.

There are three serious complications. The commonest is haemorrhage, the patient vomiting a large amount of blood. The blood is dark and granular in appearance on account of its exposure to the gastric contents; it has been called coffee-ground vomitus.

Perforation, in which the ulcer eats its way through the stomach wall, allowing the stomach or duodenal contents to escape into the peritoneum, is of the utmost seriousness because of the peritonitis which follows. It demands immediate surgery. Fortunately its symptoms, such as pain, shock, and collapse, are so striking as to call attention to itself immediately and indicate the need of assistance.

The third complication is narrowing, or stenosis, of the pylorus (the outlet of the stomach), caused by the progressive contraction of the ulcer in healing. In treating the last condition, surgery is the most valued aid, the surgeon by the operation of gastro-enterostomy making a new outlet for the stomach at its lowest point.

The treatment of simple, uncomplicated ulcer is, besides the use of alkalis already mentioned, the institution of a diet. The diet should consist of food which has the highest combining power with hydrochloric acid and the lowest irritating power.

Milk, cream, and eggs are among such articles. Lean meat, mashed potatoes, well-cooked oatmeal, and cream soups also are well tolerated. Bread, unless it be toasted or stale, sweets, fried foods, heavy vegetables, and fruits in general are very irritating.

This summarizes the approach of the orthodox to the problem of stomach ulcer. The bland diet with hourly feedings of milk may help to relieve symptoms and may therefore be desirable during the first week of an active ulcer. There is no firm evidence, however, that a bland diet speeds healing or prevents recurrence.

A more practical approach is to eliminate foods that cause the patient distress such as fatty foods, spices, fruit juices and especially pepper. Coffee, tea, cocoa and cola all stimulate acid production and are taboo. Alcohol has the same effect. There is evidence that ulcers in those who do not smoke or who stop smoking heal more rapidly.

Remember that whilst food can neutralize acid, hence the advice to eat little and often, it also stimulates acid production. Diet of the above, orthodox type is not a completely effective way of neutralizing acid, so orthodox medicine looks further to medication with drugs or by surgery. Later we shall see how sensible dieting can both heal and prevent gastric ulceration.

Antacids
Although there is no proof that antacids promote healing or prevent occurrence of peptic ulcers, they are used in orthodox therapy to give only symptomatic relief. In general there are two types of antacids:

Absorbable antacids: Sodium bicarbonate, and calcium carbonate (chalk) are the most potent antacids but they are absorbed giving high levels of sodium and calcium minerals in the body. The result is a condition called alkalosis or milk-alkali syndrome. Symptoms include nausea, weakness and headache leading, after chronic ingestion, to kidney damage. Hence soluble antacids must be used with particular caution in those whose ulcer symptoms include vomiting and haemorrhage. Those who are dehydrated because of these conditions or who suffer from high blood-pressure or kidney trouble should not take absorbable antacids. Blood calcium levels may also rise leading to calcification in the soft tissues and organs of the body.

Non-absorbable antacids: Aluminium hydroxide is commonly used as an antacid and is regarded as relatively safe yet the following side-effects may occur. Phosphate depletion can result from the binding of phosphate by aluminium in the gastro-intestinal tract. As a result, blood phosphate levels fall; the body then extracts more from the bone to make up the deficit so the bones weaken. The result is weakness, malaise and loss of appetite. Eventually the bone becomes so demineralized that breakages are relatively easy. Aluminium hydroxide may also cause constipation. Although alleged to be totally insoluble it is possible that some of the aluminium will dissolve and be absorbed. At high levels this mineral can be quite toxic.

Magnesia, which acts as magnesium hydroxide, is an effective antacid. It is often given with aluminium hydroxide to prevent the constipation induced by the latter. This is fine if the amount taken is carefully controlled but too much causes diarrhoea. As some magnesium is certainly absorbed, this treatment is not suitable for those suffering from kidney problems.

Bismuth salts were widely used in the past but are now falling into disrepute. This is largely due to lack of proof of their effectiveness, and their toxic effects which include loss of appetite, headache, malaise and skin reactions.

There is little to recommend any of the orthodox antacids in the treatment of peptic ulceration.

Anticholinergics

These drugs are given to delay emptying of the stomach which can be rapid in the case of uncomplicated duodenal ulcer. In this way antacid retention is prolonged and when taken in adequate doses, anticholinergics also diminish acid secretion. These drugs are most effective at night when regular hourly intake of antacids is impractical. Tincture of belladonna which is in this class of drugs is still widely used.

Like all drugs, however, anticholinergics provide their share of side-effects. Dry mouth, blurring of vision (or both), are not uncommon. Less common but more serious is urinary retention and glaucoma. Complete pyloric obstruction may develop in those with only partial obstruction. Anyone with oesophagitis or oesophageal ulcers cannot take anticholinergic drugs because of potential side-effects. For the same reason smokers should abstain whilst on these drugs.

Drugs that Reduce Acid Secretion
Many physicians now use therapeutic agents called histamine H_2 receptor blocking agents. These drugs act specifically by inhibiting the secretion of stomach acid. Usually the H_2 receptors in the stomach react to naturally-produced histamine by stimulating the production and secretion of hydrochloric acid. Hence by blocking these H_2 receptors in a specific manner, they no longer function and acid secretion stops.

Two such drugs are cimetidine and ranitidine. They are usually taken with each meal and at bedtime. Gastric acidity is lowered and healing of duodenal and gastric ulcers is promoted. Whilst symptoms are commonly relieved within the first week, complete healing of the ulcers may take between two and eight weeks. The usual length of treatment is four weeks. Not all ulcers are healed by these measures but the healing rate increases with length of treatment perhaps even up to 12 weeks. Unfortunately, the longer the therapy lasts the more chances there are of side-effects.

What are the likely side-effects? Diarrhoea, muscle

pain, dizziness and skin rash may occasionally occur. These are relatively mild side-effects but there are more serious ones. Impotence, lack of sperms in semen and other effects induced by the anti-sex hormone properties of cimetidine have been reported although rarely. In addition cases of acute pancreatitis and nephritis (inflammation of the kidneys) have been associated with cimetidine.

Ranitidine allegedly causes less side-effects than cimetidine but this may simply reflect its less widespread use. The chances are that as more patients are treated with ranitidine, side-effects will begin to appear.

Having established that H_2 antagonists will heal peptic ulcers in most patients, the question remains on how to prevent their recurrence. When treatment with these drugs is stopped after ulcer healing, up to eighty per cent of patients will have ulcer recurrence within one year. For this reason, the patient is often put onto maintenance therapy at a lower dose. Despite this, experience in the United Kingdom has indicated a remission rate of thirty per cent in the case of duodenal ulcers and that of twenty per cent in gastric ulcers in the first twelve months of maintenance therapy. There are however unexplained differences between patients in various countries. In duodenal ulcers recurrence during one year maintenance on ranitidine was twenty-six per cent in the UK; sixteen per cent in West Germany and a massive sixty per cent in Austria and Belgium.

There are no obvious reasons for these variations.

Age, sex, smoking habits and drug tolerance appeared to play no part. What was apparent, however, was that when maintenance therapy discontinued after one year, relapses occurred at the same rate as before treatment. The conclusion reached was that drug therapy with H_2 receptor antagonists merely suppresses the disease and does not alter its natural history.

In 1982 a World Congress of Gastroenterology, held in Stockholm, assessed the efficiency of these drugs. Whilst there was no doubt of their usefulness in healing ulcers no clear-cut decision was reached on how to prevent their recurrence in chronic disease. The choice lay between long-term maintenance therapy, with the risk of side-effects, and surgery.

One speaker suggested there were signs that the natural history of gastric and duodenal ulcers in the UK was changing to a 'less aggressive' form. Fewer patients were being presented for emergency surgery because of perforation or haemorrhage. This trend had actually started before the H_2 antagonist drugs had been introduced so there was some other, less obvious reason.

Unhappily though, it was reported that the total incidence of ulcer disease is not falling and the sad conclusion was that more and more patients would end up on long-term drug therapy. No one suggested that dietary principles could be the best cure and prevention of peptic ulcers.

One of the more serious controversies concerning cimetidine therapy was centred on the possibility of the drug causing gastric cancer. Out of 9,504 patients who had taken cimetidine, gastric cancer was diagnosed in 74. Twenty-three were diagnosed before treatment had started; 29 had gastric cancer within six months of starting therapy. Only 8 patients out of 8,994 controls (who did not receive the drug) developed gastric cancer over the same period of one year. It is possible that cimetidine had been used unwittingly to treat gastric cancer (which had been there all the time) according to those reporting the trials. It was obvious however that a possible association between cimetidine and gastric cancer had not been disproved, according to one researcher.

Liquorice

Liquorice has a soothing (or demulcent) action on the mucous membranes which is why it is used to relieve coughs and sore throats. It also has an expectorant action which helps to remove the phlegm that is often the cause of throat irritation. This demulcent property is the reason why liquorice is also a traditional remedy for peptic ulceration.

Liquorice has mild anti-inflammatory properties but in addition it can also act like the corticosteroid hormones produced in the adrenal glands. The latter are undesirable so the ideal preparation of liquorice for treating ulcers would be one that retained the demulcent and anti-inflammatory properties but reduced the hormone-like activity. Such a preparation is deglycyrrhizinised liquorice and it has found great use in healing peptic ulcers.

Another approach is to modify chemically a constituent of liquorice to produce an anti-ulcer drug. This is called carbenoxolone. Like all liquorice preparations it functions by reducing the inflammation around the ulcer and by causing the secretion of large amounts of thick protective mucus that cover the ulcer. Hence by preventing contact of hydrochloric acid with the ulcer, the mucus allows natural healing to take place. At the same time liquorice preparations stimulate cell regeneration which accelerates the rate of healing.

Because liquorice and its derivatives still retain adrenal cortex hormone-like activities, they can still exert an effect upon the minerals of the body. This leads to sodium and water retention, causing oedema. At the same time there is excessive loss of potassium in the urine along with excessive alkaline conditions in the body. High blood-pressure has been reported as well as a mild, reversible, diabetic-like condition. Heartburn can follow the ingestion of carbenoxolone in tablet form.

Liquorice and its constituents can therefore be regarded as natural agents in the successful treatment of gastric and duodenal ulcers but their use must be tempered with caution. In moderate amounts, the root can have a positive beneficial effect but at the same time its possible side-effects must be monitored since they can be detrimental. Deglycyrrhizinised liquorice appears to be the preparation of choice in terms of safety and efficacy.

Vitamin A and Gastric Ulcers

Although treatment of gastric ulcers with vitamin A can hardly be regarded as orthodox since relatively high doses are required, there is increasing interest in using this natural food constituent as a therapeutic agent. It is well known that vitamin A has a protective action on skin and mucous membranes; indeed it is one of its accepted, essential functions. For this reason it was reasoned that the vitamin had the potential for exerting a similar action against gastric ulcer. This hypothesis has been tested in a multi-centre, randomized, controlled trial of vitamin A in sixty patients with chronic gastric ulcers. The trial took place in Hungary and was reported in *The Lancet* towards the end of 1982.

There were three groups of patients. One group was treated only with antacids; the second group received similar antacids with the addition of 150,000IU of vitamin A daily; the third group were given the same doses of vitamin A and antacids daily with the addition of cyproheptadine, an antihistamine drug, also daily. All patients were treated for four weeks. Ulcer sizes were measured before and after treatment in each case.

All ulcers were reduced to a significant degree but those patients receiving vitamin A experienced a significantly greater reduction in size than those treated just with antacids. The authors concluded that 'a beneficial effect of vitamin A has been indicated in the prevention and treatment of stress ulcers in patients'.

No simple clinical trial is accepted by the medical fraternity as conclusive until it has been repeated with similar success. The above trial was conducted on patients with stress-induced gastric ulcers. It was therefore repeated on patients suffering from chronic and recurrent gastric ulcers and reported in the *International Journal of Tissue Reactions* in 1983. The second trial was a randomized, prospective study of sixty patients with chronic gastric ulcer. One group received antacids only; the second group were given antacids plus 50,000IU vitamin A three times daily and the third group received the same medication as the second group but with the addition of an antihistamine drug. As before, treatment was continued for four weeks. The number of patients with completely healed ulcers was higher in the groups which received vitamin A. In addition, the reduction in ulcer size was greater in patients who were given vitamin A. The authors concluded that 'vitamin A has a beneficial effect in the process of ulcer healing in patients with chronic gastric ulcer'.

One pleasing aspect of both trials was the complete lack of toxic side-effects despite the relatively high intakes of vitamin A. They suggest that 150,000IU daily for four weeks is a dose of the vitamin easily tolerated over this period. The excellent response is an indication of natural treatment. On the other hand, as we shall see later, these results also suggest that prevention of gastric ulceration can be brought about by an adequate intake of this vitamin throughout life.

Gastric ulcers can be thought of as a pre-cancerous state and significant negative correlation has been reported between body levels of vitamin A and the development of various cancers. In other words low levels of the vitamin appear to be found regularly in cases of cancer of the lung, bladder and skin. The results of these two trials indicate a possible role for gastric protection in the prevention of the development of gastric cancer from gastric ulcer.

The Use of Cabbage Juice

Professor Garnet Cheney, of the Stanford Medical School, California, has had success with cabbage juice in the treatment of stomach ulcers. He says that it is the Vitamin C factor in the juice which has such powerful healing qualities. This may only be partly true since the same researcher reported a unique factor, called vitamin U, in cabbage leaves and other vegetables. This has been called the anti-ulcer vitamin. Vitamin U has been isolated from cabbage leaves and has also been produced by chemical synthesis. It is known under the trade names of *Caboagin-U, Epadyn-U, Vitas U* and *Ardesyl*.

Cabbage juice is quite a pleasant drink, but the processing really requires an electric juicer, and these are expensive. It would be wise to regard cabbage juice as a supplementary factor in the cure of stomach ulcer, and not to place the onus of cure upon it. Whatever the virtues of cabbage juice, it is not a substitute for the curative and preventative principles set out in this book. Most cabbages are raised on soils fertilized with chemical manures and this reduces their vitamin content and nutritional value.

Garlic

Oil of garlic has remarkable healing properties and

has been used in Europe and Asia for centuries.
Garlic is a cleanser and kills the unfriendly bacteria
B. coli in the large intestine, thereby lightening the
duties of the liver and spleen. Garlic improves the
appetite, reduces blood tension and helps to prevent
thrombosis. It is excellent in respiratory troubles;
is highly regarded as a nerve tonic and remedies
flatulence and diarrhoea. It is recognized as a most
valuable intestinal antiseptic. Garlic capsules, each
containing three minims of pure oil of garlic, are
readily available.

Herbal Remedies
We have discussed already one herbal remedy for
peptic ulcers, that is, liquorice. In addition, however,
there are other traditional remedies for gastric
conditions and one of the better established and
more effective ones is althaea root, otherwise
known as marshmallow root. Its main active constituent is mucilage but it also contains sterols,
asparagin and lecithin, all of which contribute to its
beneficial effect. Marshmallow has a demulcent
action combined with an emollient or softening
and soothing effect. For this reason the root is
recommended for gastritis and enteritis but its
specific indications are gastric and duodenal ulcers.
The usual dose is between 2 and 5g of the dried root
three times daily. A more effective preparation is a
combination of marshmallow with symphytum.

Symphytum: This is more commonly known as
comfrey and it is active in either the root or leafy
form. Both have a demulcent action that is due to

their content of mucilage, allantoin, symphitine and echimidine. They have found use in the treatment of gastric and duodenal ulcers. The usual dose of dried root or dried leaves is 2-4g or 4-8g respectively, taken at the rate of three doses per day.

Slippery Elm Bark: Also known as ulmus, it is another rich source of mucilage which explains its beneficial actions as a demulcent and emollient. Unlike most herbal remedies it contains significant amounts of starch which contributes to its food properties. Specifically it is used to help heal gastric and duodenal ulcers. The powdered bark is usually extracted with water at the rate of 1 part bark to 8 parts water. The liquid (4-16cc) is drunk three times daily. There are however many commercial preparations of dried bark extract that are more convenient to take.

Failure of Ulcer Operations

With the exception of urgent surgical operations to repair the damage where an ulcer has eaten a hole right through to the peritoneum, ulcer operations have a record of failure. To cut out an ulcer and draw the wall of the stomach together, cannot possibly be described as a 'cure'. But it can be described as a very dangerous intrusion into an area of the body that Nature, in her wisdom, has carefully and hermetically sealed, and is often followed by serious results for the patient. If the patient recovers and goes on in the same old dietetic way, further ulcers will occur, and what then? More operations?

Dr Richard Harrison (USA) expressed this view: 'A man or woman who has stomach ulcer is sick all over. It is utterly ridiculous and dangerous to treat a stomach ulcer by localised medication or by surgical removal.'

Dr Walter C. Alvarez, of the Mayo Clinic, said: 'If the patient is worrisome and temperamental, operation is probably useless.'

What pain-racked, nerve-racked ulcer sufferer is *not* worrisome and temperamental? By this time he is beside himself with suffering. Dr James Brown, in a treatise on the subject, points out that even after an operation, 'treatment of the complaint has only begun'.

In his book *Peptic Ulcer*, Dr T. L. Cleave states that every year 30,000 human stomachs are removed in operating theatres in the United Kingdom. After praising the skill of the surgeons, Dr Cleave points out that the operation carries liabilities. There is loss of energy and the patient may be compared to 'a bird that has lost a handful of feathers from one wing'. Another liability never usually mentioned, says Dr Cleave, is that the original cause of the trouble continues to operate and 'other diseases may supervene in the future'.

Diet Supersedes Surgery
Dr B. P. Allinson, a member of the Royal College of Surgeons, in the course of a lecture given in London on unnecessary operative surgery said:

The question arises as to how much abdominal

surgery is justified, and here again I personally am no doubt apt to form any conclusions from the failures I have seen, though, speaking in general, I think that most surgery that is performed for ulcers should not be performed. There is much surgery for ulceration, and I see a great many of the failures of this surgery, more especially of what are called short-circuit operations. In these cases one has to deal with an additional disability in the form of the operative interference that has taken place.

I think that adequate natural methods, principally dietetic methods, can deal with digestive ulceration, especially with chronic digestive ulceration, much more satisfactorily than surgery can, and in this case I would especially emphasise the non-toxic diet, that is, avoiding all poisons, especially tea, coffee, tobacco, alcohol, and all flesh foods.

On a diet of that description not only do these ulcers heal but they remain healed which is important, because one of the surgeon's dicta in the subject is: 'Oh, it is all very well; you may heal an ulcer with a diet, but it will come back again, and then an emergency will arise'.

That again, as I say, is true within the surgeon's own experience, but I have dealt with quite a large number of ulcers, principally duodenal ulcers, which are more common than gastric ulcers, and they have healed and they have remained healed.

I have had two relapses out of a number, but even in those cases the ulcers healed again after the relapse and remained healed. If the surgeon were to know that a proper diet would heal the ulcers perfectly, as long as the individual adhered to it, then perhaps he would modify his view about the necessity of surgery.

It is important to remember also the consequences

of partial or total removal of the stomach by surgery. The operation results in loss of hydrochloric acid production; loss of stomach digestive enzymes; loss of intrinisic factor secretion. The latter, as we have seen, will prevent the absorption of vitamin B_{12}, so pernicious anaemia may result. This is why regular injections of vitamin B_{12} are essential to anyone who has had a partial or complete gastrectomy. The consequences of lack of hydrochloric acid production have already been discussed.

Surgery's Attack on the Ulcer

A development in operative surgery for ulcers is to sever the vagus nerve. This is called vagotomy. The theory behind this new and desperate exploration into the abdominal cavity is as follows. Some ulcer cases are nervy, worrisome, restless types. While they are in this state, the gastric juice is constantly flowing, due to the fact that the vagus nerve connects the stomach with the brain. If the stomach could be disconnected from the brain, by cutting the vagus nerve, then the stomach would not be affected by the state of the patient's brain, and his worries, etc.

That is the theory of the surgery, but it is not now a common approach in Britain and the USA to attack the problem of stomach ulcers by severing the vagus nerve. The more advanced medical man, who puts his faith in sound nutrition, views this surgical intrusion into the human body with alarm. He points out that the vagus nerve not only connects the stomach to the brain, but supplies branches to the heart, lungs, throat and abdomen.

To sever this vitally important nerve may have serious repercussions on the sympathetic nervous system which controls these organs. It is a clumsy, even dangerous method of attempting to control overactivity on the part of the nervous system and the flow of gastric fluids. It is significant that the usual sensational claims of success have not been made in the case of this type of operation.

Where Orthodox Treatment Fails

Orthodox medical treatment is notorious for its failure to cure ulcers in the digestive tract because:

1. It makes no attempt to correct the dietetic errors of the patient.

2. It resorts to a 'soft, bland diet' which, while temporarily coating the ulcer, is in its nature constipating and deficient in vitamins and minerals. Indeed, fresh fruits and raw salad vegetables are not permitted because they might 'irritate' the ulcer! Orthodox medicine quite overlooks the fact that these sores can only be healed by raising the purity and tone of the blood-stream, and by maintaining this purity and tone permanently. It was the absence of vitamins and minerals that largely caused the ulcer in the first place. No ulcer is likely to form in the digestive tract of a person whose blood-stream had been consistently fed on foods rich in vitamins and minerals.

3. To resort to antacid powders, bicarbonate of soda and milk of magnesia to supply alkalines is just another example of the educated ignorance so

common in orthodox medical practice.

4. Surgery is rarely necessary for the narrowing of the pylorus caused by an ulcer. This condition rarely fails to respond to a diet of well-diluted fruit juices or vegetable juices, which have an alkaline reaction in the body.

6

Views on Causes and Cures

Orthodox medical men put far too much emphasis on worry and the strains of modern life as the main causes of ulcers. Nevertheless doctors do get the impression that peptic ulcers are commonest in tense, anxious people. Nervous tension makes them worse so sufferers are advised to calm themselves down if they can. What is certain is that smoking, even though it may help calm some people, will make peptic ulcers worse.

Sir Robert McCarrison, who was for some years medical officer among the Hunza in Northern India, failed to find one case of stomach ulcer, kidney disease or heart disease among those people over a period of nine years. The Hunza live on vegetables, cheese, fruit, milk and coarse grain mostly, with meat as a luxury once in a while. These people also live calm unstressful lives without the problems and pace of modern civilization and this too may be a factor, along with that of their diet, in keeping them free of the scourge of peptic ulcers.

Women and Children Now Ulcer Victims
The following excerpts from a cable from New

York, published in the press of 29 January 1961, are of interest:

'Stomach ulcers, once considered an exclusively male disease, are now attacking women and children in alarming numbers. U.S. research figures this week showed that the number of women sufferers had risen by about 350 per cent in the past 20 years. A British doctor found that nine of a family of 13 had duodenal ulcers. Doctors were fast revising old theories about what foods an ulcer sufferer should eat or avoid.

'American doctors are staging an all-out attack on the ailment that in the U.S. alone costs the nation £222 million a year in medical bills and loss of work time. Authorities point out that there is a growing number of female ulcer sufferers due to the increased commitments of the working woman. "Today's woman is competing actively with man outside her home, while inside she has become a full partner in marriage, sharing the decisions that affect her family's future," a noted psychiatrist said this week . . .

'In a recent British project, doctors discovered that . . . dieting with bland foods does not increase the rate of healing of peptic ulcers . . .'

At the Mayo Clinic in Rochester, Minnesota, 2,000 patients being treated for arthritis with aspirin-type medications were found to have four times as many ulcers as the other patients. Other doctors have observed that large amounts of aspirin taken by ulcer sufferers coincide with bleeding.

'A British study found more ulcers among truck drivers and baggage clerks than among professional men. On the lowest social level of unskilled labourers, the men's ulcer rate was found to be 116 per cent of the national average. On the highest, the rate was only 48 per cent.'

An Ulcer Specialist Supports Our Views
Fortunately, there is a growing, if small, percentage of medical practitioners who are leading the profession in the new and sounder approach to the problem of acidity and stomach ulcer.

One of these is the famous Scottish doctor, Dr Fyfe Robertson, who was himself a sufferer from stomach ulcer for years. He is a recognized authority on the subject and has cured hundreds of very bad cases, including himself. Dr Fyfe Robertson has no hesitation in saying that it is the 'degradation of food' during the past century that has given rise to the alarming increase in stomach ulcer. He explains that the degradation of food has been due to '"Scientific" farming, which alters the nature of things that grow in the soil—by the use of artificial fertilisers and sprays to kill plant diseases and pests; and injections to fight animal diseases. Food-processing methods which rob foods of most of their virtue—in the case of white flour, of almost everything except starch. Use of preservatives, "improvers", colouring and flavouring agents, of artificial chemical substances which are often poisonous. Loss of nutritive value through increasing staleness of foods. In spite of better transport, many foodstuffs are older and staler when they reach the consumer than they were 50 years ago.

'And freezing, gas storage, chemical preserving

have advantages—but they do not improve foods. The nostalgia of the elderly for the foods of their youth is justified; they were fresher, tastier and more wholesome, because they were whole foods.

'Apologists for modern food practices excuse them individually because their effects, individually, are so small. But cumulatively they are enormous.'

The Menace of Preservative Poisons

Dr Robertson continues: 'Consider a diet including dyed, frozen, gassed, canned, chemically preserved and flavoured foods; eggs from hens unnaturally fed and kept; stale fish; stale vegetables often grown by suspect methods; processed cheese instead of original real cheese; "full fruit" jam preserved with sulphur dioxide and chemically dyed; white sugar, vitaminless and consumed in over-large quantities; cereal foods heat-treated before the consumer gets them. "A man is what he eats", so the old saying goes. Would you rule out the possibility that these things, operating daily for years and in the unborn child, may be the cause of bodily changes and damage? We have largely abolished the dirt disease, but the most significant medical fact today is the alarming increase in chronic degenerative diseases. Now these degenerative diseases are rarely found among people, primitive or civilized, who eat fresh, whole, unprocessed, naturally grown foods. The kind of food changes outlined here have taken place in most industrialised countries at about the same time with the rise in ulcers, particularly duodenal.'

What One Experiment Proved

'Brilliant physician Sir Robert McCarrison, one of the greatest figures in the science of nutrition, proved that differences in the physique and disease incidence among India's people could be directly related to food differences.

'Feeding rats from the same stock for 700 days (equal to 50 human years) on three human diets selected from different areas, he found that those given the worst in protein, vitamins, minerals, and over-rich in starch suffered most in health. Of the rats worst fed 29 per cent had duodenal and gastric ulcers. Those fed on a 'natural' balanced diet had no ulcers.

'When in another experiment McCarrison fed one group on the best diet and another on one of the kinds of foods eaten by the British poor, he had to segregate the "British" rats to stop them eating each other. Post-mortems of all rats after 190 days (equal to 16 human years) showed gastric ulcers, gastritis, enteritis, colitis in the "British" group, but none in the properly fed group. Even the psychiatrist must concede the significance of results like these. And the ulcer victim, drinking his alkalis, anxiously eating his miserable diet, coping with nausea, hiding the pain that grips and gnaws, fearing the meal his hunger pain makes so desirable, may wonder why findings so convincing as McCarrison's have not led to a new approach to this problem. Basically orthodox medical treatment has not changed in many years. There have, of course, been fashions—many.'

Old Treatment Still Used

Dr Robertson continues: 'Sippy's milk and alkali
diet, introduced in 1915, still holds the field, with
refinements, with orthodox medical men. This is
based on the belief that ulcers are caused by the
stomach's hydrochloric acid—that the patient's
own digestive juice is digesting the protein of his
stomach wall, which is probably true, but as the
"last link" of the chain-causes. The aim therefore is
to absorb it with chemical absorbents, to use it up
with frequent meals.

'Since it is believed that the high stomach activity
often found in ulcer cases aggravates damage and
pain, drugs to reduce muscular activity are also
given. The diet mainstay is milk, with eggs second,
and the drill is frequent meals. Some doctors give
foods or alkalis or both every two hours. The latest
fad is the sucking all day of alkali-loaded milk
tablets, since alkalis (owing to stomach emptying)
do not act for more than about 15 minutes.

'No roughage is allowed—not even the tiniest, as
it is believed that pain is caused by food passing
over the ulcer. If the diet is bland, it is also
unappetising and dreary. The prohibitions are
immense, quite often unnecessary and psychologically disastrous. Surgical treatment has had
many fashions, the tendency being to more and
more drastic methods. A new technique, severance
of the nerves controlling stomach movement and
acid secretion, is already discredited. Surgery has
improved and for some conditions it is essential,
but it is not now so lightly recommended.'

Stomach Ulcers—A Deficiency Ailment

Dr D. T. Quigley in *The National Malnutrition* wrote: 'The first treatment for stomach ulcer which attained any great attention by the medical profession was the so-called Sippy treatment. This treatment consisted in neutralizing the highly acid condition of the stomach with chalk and other alkalines, but it also included hourly feedings of milk or cream and orange juice. Sippy knew nothing whatever of vitamins, and perhaps never thought of such a thing as mineral deficiency in this class of disease, but through a fortuitous accident his treatment provided the patient with calcium and also with the vitamins contained in butter fat, milk, and orange juice.

'This treatment supplies only a part of the whole deficiency needs of a person with this type of disease, but it was so great an improvement over the deficiency diets which produced the disease that many patients were temporarily cured. Sippy and the others of his time did not recognize the fact that the patient needed not a temporary treatment, but a permanent one. They did not recognize the fact that the ulcers were due to dietary deficiences and that the patients must be put on a correct diet for the rest of their lives. They assumed that the patient was consuming a normal diet, and that the ulcer was due to some mysterious and unexplainable happening which in some way was connected with the production of too much acid in the stomach. We now know that the acid is the defence mechanism. It is the only mechanism the stomach has for fighting back against irritations from without. The person suffering with this kind of disease always has some degree of scurvy. The scurvy has produced bad teeth and infected gums. The bad teeth and infected gums have caused pus to be swallowed into the stomach, sometimes at the rate of about a teaspoonful every hour. The swallowing of pus produces local irritation. The irritation calls out the increased stomach secretion. Continuation of the irritation results in an increase of hydrochloric acid, leading eventually to ulceration. These happenings cover a period of years, and by the time the ulcer appears in the stomach or duodenum the whole gastro-intestinal tract is diseased and along with it the liver duct and gall bladder. The ulcer is a focal breakdown in a completely diseased gastro-intestinal canal.

'On the clinical side, many internists and some surgeons have come to consider vitamin C as a cure for stomach ulcers. Here they are recognizing a truth, but only a part of the whole truth—lack of vitamin C is undoubtedly one of the predominant causes of stomach ulcer. A complete treatment would mean a treatment with all other vitamins and minerals lacking in the individual's diet, as well as with vitamin C.'

Gayelord Hauser on the Cure of Stomach Ulcer
Gayelord Hauser, American nutritional scientist, confirmed most of the conclusions arrived at in this book when he wrote in *Diet Does It!*:

'In few instances has the diet used in the correction of disease been so disgracefully inadequate as that given to persons suffering from ulcers of the stomach or duodenum. The Sippy diet, which consists of taking milk and cream every two hours, was first used when the science of nutrition was unknown. Yet it is still in general use. The principles upon which it was built, however, are as unsound today as they were then. An ulcer is nothing more than a sore in the wall of the stomach or intestine. The normal stomach secretes strong hydrochloric acid from which the stomach and intestinal walls are usually protected by a covering of thick mucus. The ulcerated spot, however, cannot produce mucus by which to protect itself; yet the ulcer cannot heal readily with strong acid pouring over it.'

'The reason for recommending that an ulcer patient drink milk and cream every two hours is that milk combines with hydrochloric acid and cream inhibits its flow; thus acid is kept from the ulcer until it has a chance to heal. The person who wishes to recover from an ulcer should drink a glass of milk every two hours or, if the pain is severe, half a glass every hour. If the patient is overweight, skim milk can be used. The difficulty with a milk diet, however, is that it is inadequate in almost all vitamins and in iron and copper. Cases have been reported in the *Journal of the American Medical Association* of people who have developed both scurvy and beriberi, diseases caused by an almost total lack of vitamin C and B, while living on a milk diet. The milk and cream diet, therefore, must be modified in order to make it adequate, to increase rapid healing, and to prevent the recurrence of ulcers.

Hauser on Vitamins for Ulcer

'Two new methods used in the correction of ulcer have met with marked success. One is the giving of massive doses of vitamin A, which maintains the health of mucous membrane lining the walls of the stomach and intestine. The other treatment is that of giving 1,000 milligrams of vitamin C daily for three days in the form of 100 milligram tablets; the amount is increased by 100 milligrams daily until the dosage reaches 2,000 milligrams; this amount should then be continued indefinitely. This large amount of Vitamin C stimulates the formation of scar tissue and causes the ulcer to heal rapidly. Citrus juices are usually avoided because of the citric acid they contain, but vegetable juices, especially carrot juice, can be used freely. (Citrus juices can, however, be used if well diluted with water.) These two methods are excellent and are to be recommended to anyone with an active ulcer. Even with whole milk and ample amounts of vitamins A and C, the diet is still markedly inadequate. The person with an ulcer must obtain the vitamins of the B family. At least a half cup of short-cooked wheatgerm should be eaten each morning, and a tablespoonful of powdered brewer's yeast stirred into milk should be taken after each meal. All liquids should be drunk through a straw. (This is to avoid swallowing air which may result in flatulence.) Iron and copper can be obtained from a serving of wheatgerm.'

The Bioflavonoids and Stomach Ulcers

Recent research indicates that improved healing

follows when vitamin C is taken in conjunction with the bioflavonoid complex. A special tablet is available which contains 100mg of the bioflavonoid complex, 95mg vitamin C and 5mg rose hips. These tablets can be taken for stomach ulcers as well as, or in replacement of vitamin C tablets. We suggest that a bioflavonoid and vitamin C tablet be taken twice daily, after meals, in addition to the vitamin C tablets already listed.

'When Cured, Keep On Vital Diet', said Hauser
'Fruit and vegetables need be puréed only if they are not well tolerated otherwise. Thorough chewing is essential. After the ulcer has healed it is of extreme importance to continue the Vital Diet indefinitely to maintain healthy scar tissue. Otherwise an ulcer will quickly recur. I believe it is correct to say that if a Vital Diet is maintained, day after day and year after year, infections and the many resulting handicaps will be a thing of the past.'

7

Thirteen Curative Principles

Having dealt earlier in this book with the causes of
indigestion and stomach ulcer, the curative principles will naturally consist of not doing those very
things which singly, or together, caused the trouble.
The first principle of curing any ailment is to stop
causing it. To put the matter more positively, we
have summarized the advice given by the world's
leading medical scientists in regard to the cure of
indigestion, ulcers, and stomach troubles generally
into thirteen simple principles, which any sufferer
can understand and apply:

Eat Less
(1) Eat much less than you were in the habit of
eating. Eat simply. Make a meal of one course—one
kind of mild fruit, or salad, or lightly cooked
vegetables. (Study the Science of Life book *Eating
for Health*).

Take Supplements
(2) Build up your starved nervous organization by
systematically taking the B$_1$, B complex and calcium
tablets recommended in the diet for stomach
ulcers.

Protein and Ulcers: Experiments with laboratory animals have disclosed that if they are kept on a diet deficient in protein, one hundred per cent of them develop ulcers of the duodenum or stomach. Similarly, persons with stomach or duodenal ulcers are often found to have lived on diets lacking in protein. Even when stomach ulcers in such persons have healed, they soon recur if too little protein is included in the daily diet. Having developed a stomach ulcer, it cannot be healed quickly, however, merely by increasing one's daily intake of protein. Why? Because all protein foods stimulate the flow of the gastric juices, which contain a powerful acid (hydrochloric) needed to digest proteins. This acid erodes and irritates the raw surface of the stomach ulcer, giving rise to pain. The first thing to be done therefore is to help nature to establish a protective coating over the ulcer and thereby expedite the healing process. To do this it is necessary to cut down one's intake of protein foods to a minimum for several weeks. This gives the ulcerous surface a respite from the irritation set up by the acid mentioned. No more than two or three ounces of cheese should be taken daily during this period. It is best to omit meat altogether for the first two weeks, as meat is inferior to cheese in nutritional qualities and is not so easily digested. Wheatgerm can be used later and may be short cooked if desired.

Cheese: Cheese, as we have seen, is a more valuable form of protein than meat and has more energy value and nourishment. In addition, cheese contains lactic acid which aids digestion and is rich in calcium, essential to strong nerves and healthy tissue. Packeted cheese is generally processed and it is therefore advisable to purchase unprocessed block cheese.

Take Alkaline-forming Foods
(3) See that approximately 80 per cent of your food consists of alkaline-forming foods (fruit, raw salad vegetables, cooked vegetables, milk and dried fruits) and only 20 per cent of the acid-forming foods (meat, fish, eggs, cheese, bread, concentrated starches and sugary foods). Not alkaline powders but alkaline foods and diluted fruit juices possess the secret of neutralizing excessive acidity in the stomach, and maintaining the proper acid/alkaline balance in the blood. That is a simple, easy-to-remember principle of first-class health.

Avoid Incompatible Feeding
(4) Avoid incompatible feeding in the following ways:

(a) Don't eat a protein and a concentrated starch or sugary food at the same meal;
(b) Don't eat a concentrated starch food (such as white bread and potatoes) and an acid fruit at the same meal;
(c) Don't eat a milk pudding or drink milk on top of a meat meal;
(d) Don't eat raw and cooked vegetables or raw and stewed fruits at the same meal.

In the case of (a), (b), and (c) protein foods require

an acid solution for their digestion. They are primarily digested by the gastric juice secreted in the stomach. All other foods require an alkaline solution for their digestion. This is secreted in the mouth and is mixed with the food in the saliva. A sick stomach cannot be both acid and alkaline at the same time. This is a difficult enough feat for a healthy stomach to achieve.

Make Good Vitamin Deficiencies

(5) All vitamin and mineral deficiencies must be made good and maintained as a regular routine of life. The following vitamins, which are the great healing agents for stomach ulcers, and also ulcers of the duodenum and pylorus, should be taken consistently before each meal, three times daily. They can all be taken together.

   1 Vitamin E tablet or capsule (100mg)
   1 Vitamin A tablet or capsules (2,500 IU*)
   1 Vitamin B$_1$ tablet (10mg)
   1 Vitamin B complex tablet (10mg strength)
   1 Vitamin C tablet (250mg)
   2 calcium tablets, white (75mg each of calcium)
   *(If vitamin A capsules are used instead of tablets, these should be taken after meals.)

Once daily, a pantothenic acid tablet should be taken (at least 100mg). Where the diet is rich in calcium foods—milk, cream, cheese—the calcium tablets may be omitted. Such a diet would include 2 pints (1.1 litres) of milk and 4oz (115g) of cheese daily.

Extra B vitamins are needed for a variety of

reasons. Persistent use of antacids, for example, particularly amongst older people can lead to impaired absorption of vitamin B_1 with subsequent low body levels of the vitamin. It is important therefore to take vitamin B_1 supplements to ensure an adequate intake. Younger people are not immune either as they too can suffer from persistent dyspepsia. One consequence of too little vitamin B_1 is constipation so taking supplements of the vitamin whilst suffering from one gastro-intestinal complaint can prevent another.

Vitamin B_2 is needed to maintain healthy mucous membranes and it can have a preventative and curative effect on those suffering from mouth ulcers. There is no doubt that sometimes the type of person likely to suffer from peptic ulcers is also the type to develop mouth ulcers. Hence it is sound supplementation to ensure an adequate daily intake of vitamin B_2, also in those liable to gastric and duodenal ulcers.

When nicotinamide, or vitamin B_3, is deficient, one of the common symptoms is gastro-intestinal upsets characterized by nausea, vomiting and sometimes inflammation of the mouth and digestive tract. These symptoms, as we have seen, are also associated with gastric and duodenal ulceration so a daily supplement of nicotinamide is a useful insurance policy.

Pantothenic acid is a B vitamin that is needed in the production of anti-stress hormones. Hence if the individual is the stressed, nervous or overwrought type, the result can be an increased tendency for them to develop gastric or duodenal ulcers. Adequate pantothenic acid and, indeed, vitamin C, also will at least ensure that anti-stress hormone production is not deficient and the tendency to produce ulcers is lessened.

Need for Fat
When insufficient fat is included in the diet, foods leave the stomach fairly rapidly and the walls of the stomach are then exposed to the action of strong hydrochloric acid for lengthy periods. We advise that a little fatty food be eaten at every meal and after meals, a teaspoonful of olive oil be taken.

Vitamin A
Quite apart from the value of vitamin A in building a healthy lining to the stomach, intestines, throat and lungs, it is vitally important for resistance to all infections. In addition though, as we have seen, high doses of this vitamin can actually heal ulcers. It is therefore quite possible that adequate intakes daily may help prevent ulceration in the first place.

How Vitamin C Heals Ulcers
Vitamin C strengthens connective tissue and the walls of the blood vessels, both of which are essential in the healing of stomach ulcers. Dr John Marks of Downing College, Cambridge, England has written in his *Guide to the Vitamins* that in gastrointestinal disturbances vitamin C deficiency may arise through impaired absorption. The beneficial effect of vitamin C upon wound healing makes it essential that adequate amounts be administered in all cases of gastric and duodenal ulcers especially

as 'ulcer diets' are usually deficient in the vitamin.

Some advanced doctors in the USA are getting remarkably good results with 1500 milligrams of vitamin C daily. However, the important thing to do is to heal the ulcer as quickly as possible. The quantity mentioned—1500 milligrams of vitamin C daily—is obtained by taking six 250 milligram vitamin C tablets daily.

What Vitamin E Does

Animal experiments have indicated that when subjected to stress, those given large amounts of vitamin E developed far fewer and less serious ulcers than those who received nothing but a standard diet. For example, in one experiment reported in the *American Journal of Clinical Nutrition* in 1972, Dr G. F. Solomon and his colleagues compared rats that were subjected to stressful conditions. One group received 50mg vitamin E orally twice a day along with one meal; the other group received just the one meal. After 12 days, the unsupplemented rats developed 78 per cent more ulceration than those receiving vitamin E.

It is possible that vitamin E can have a sparing effect in vitamin A deficiency. As long ago as 1946, Dr J. L. Jensen published in the journal *Science* his finding that vitamin E prevented stomach ulcers in rats receiving very low amounts of vitamin A. Later, a follow-up experiment was reported by Dr T. L. Harris and associates in the *Proceedings of the Society for Experimental Biology and Medicine* in 1947. Forty young rats were placed on a diet deficient in both vitamins A and E, which is known to produce ulcers. After two weeks, all rats were given vitamin A but only half of them received vitamin E. After seven weeks the rats were examined for stomach lesions. One half, those on the high vitamin A, low vitamin E diet, had developed stomach ulcers. Not one animal in the group receiving vitamin E showed any sign of ulceration. We know that vitamin E strengthens muscular tissue and improves blood circulation. However, it also appears to help vitamin A function, in part by protecting it, so perhaps it is not surprising that vitamin E has remarkable healing properties in ulcerous conditions.

Other Curative Measures

The remaining curative measures are self-explanatory. They are:

(6) Avoid mixed, indiscriminate feeding.

(7) If you cannot eat a meal leisurely, in a state of mental and physical relaxation, it is better not to eat at all. The wise patient will cultivate the habit of having fifteen minutes' quiet repose before and after every meal, and he will have his meals at regular intervals.

(8) Omit all condiments.

(9) Cut out sugar. Never use saccharine. Substitute honey. By gradually reducing the amount of sweetening you like, you can easily cultivate a taste for unsweetened foods in a matter of weeks.

(10) With the introduction of such foods as wheat-germ, and the vitamins, you should have regular and adequate bowel movements without the use of

laxative pills or purgatives. Cut them out because they are dangerous irritants. If you still have any bowel trouble, take one or two teaspoons of molasses in warm water before going to bed.

(11) As we have seen, antacid and other alkaline powders are an unsound way of neutralizing stomach acidity. They offer a temporary respite from pain at the cost of making the condition worse. There is only one sound and certain way to cure excessive stomach acidity. Restore the proper acid-alkaline balance in your blood-stream by seeing that your diet consists of approximately 80 per cent of alkaline-forming foods and only about 20 per cent of acid-forming foods (see page 110 for details). If, in addition, you feed compatibly and generally follow the curative principles recommended, stomach acidity will plague you no more.

(12) Slow down the tempo of your life and cultivate the almost lost art of relaxation. Men who relax live longer—and it doesn't merely seem longer! To relax successfully you must make conscious and objective effort. Relax in the sun every day when possible, for fifteen to thirty minutes. The sun helps one to relax perfectly. It also helps to build good nerves—and good health. And make sure you get eight to nine hours' sleep at a regular retiring hour. The body repairs itself during sleep. There is no substitute for sleep, which Shakespeare described in *Macbeth* as 'Chief nourisher in life's feast'.

(13) Finally, by generally building up the health you also build up the resistance of the blood to noxious bacteria and virus invasions. This is of vital

importance to the ulcer sufferer because while his resistance is low, an ulcer is a breeding ground for harmful bacteria.

Dietary Suggestions for Treating Ulcers, Gastritis and Hiatus Hernia

The principle of these dietary suggestions is to buffer gastric acidity by providing several meals per day of palatable, non-irritating foods.

Foods that are allowed include milk, cream, prepared cereals (farina, cream of wheat, strained oatmeal, puffed rice, whole wheatflakes), gelatine, soup, potatoes, rice, polyunsaturated margarine, wholemeal bread, eggs, cooked fruits and vegetables, bananas (at certain times, see later), fruit juices, very lean meats (beef, lamb), fresh fish, cream or cottage cheese, custards, tapioca, rice or cornstarch pudding, plain cake made with wholewheat flours. Multivitamin supplementation is essential.

Foods to avoid include fried or highly seasoned food, spices, carbonated beverages, coffee, alcohol, meat broths, strong cheeses, coarse cereals or bread, raw fruits and vegetables (in the early stages of the complaint), rich desserts, pastry, nuts, olives and popcorn.

A typical sample bland diet is as follows:

Breakfast: Wheatgerm with milk or sugar; egg, bread with polyunsaturated margarine; jelly; milk; strained fruit or fresh fruit juices.

Lunch: Clear soup; lean meat; potato, rice or noodles; bread with polyunsaturated margarine; jelly; milk; strained fruit juices.

Dinner: Lean meat, fish or fowl; potato; two strained cooked vegetables; bread with polyunsaturated margarine; dessert; milk; strained fruit juices.

(Milk may be taken at any time between meals and at bedtime.)

Gastro-intestinal Tract Irritability

This diet is taken to spare the gastro-intestinal tract by frequent small feedings of easily digested low-residue nutrients. The content is sugars, milk, eggs, lean beef, lamb, fish or chicken, cooked refined cereals, enriched bread, polyunsaturated margarine, cottage or cream cheese, strained cooked fruits and vegetables (or juices), potatoes, bouillon, broth, clear soups, pasta, custards, dairy ice-cream, gelatine, milk puddings, plain cake.

For a low residue diet it is important to avoid highly seasoned or fried foods (to prevent irritation), whole or raw fruits and vegetables, wholegrain cereals and bread, bran, corn, dried legumes, port, excessive fat, nuts, jams and marmalade.

Strict Diet for Ulcer Sufferers

When ulcer symptoms are severe the following diet inhibits and neutralizes gastric acid secretions and relieves pain.

Step 1. Give 3oz (90ml) of cold or chilled skimmed milk or milk drinks hourly between 7 am and 9 pm.

The drink may also be continued throughout the night if there is difficulty in sleeping.

Step 2. Continue the hourly milk feedings and gradually add egg and finely-ground cereal so that the patient is receiving egg instead of milk at 7 am and 7 pm. At 10 am, 1 pm and 4 pm, 3 oz (85g) of cooked cereal should replace the milk.

Step 3. A soft diet that provides essential nutrients in a form that is low in residue, well tolerated and easily digested. Suitable foods are strained soups and vegetables; fine wheat, corn or rice cereals; breads; cooked fruit (without skin or seeds); ripe bananas, grapefruit or orange sections; fresh fruit juices; potatoes; rice; ground beef; fish, fowl; eggs; cottage or cream cheese; milk; custards; gelatine; tapioca; milk puddings; ice-cream; plain cake.

Supplementary iron and other minerals, preferably as the well-absorbed amino acid chelates plus multivitamin supplements, are essential in these diets if the strict regime is continued for an extended time. Foods that must be avoided include raw fruits and vegetables, coarse breads and cereals, rich desserts, strong spices, veal, pork, all fried foods, nuts and raisins.

Diet and Vitamin Therapy for Peptic Ulcers and Acidity

Here is a suggested diet for stomach ulcer and acidity:

FIRST DAY

On rising: Glass of milk (to be sipped slowly, not drunk) with four B complex vitamin tablets.

Before breakfast: 1 vitamin A tablet, 1 B_1 (10mg) tablet, 1 B complex tablet (10mg potency), 1 vitamin C tablet (250mg), 1 vitamin E tablet or capsule (100mg), 1 teaspoonful of olive oil.

Breakfast: Three or more dessertspoons of a reputable brand of wheatgerm, and as much milk as you can tolerate without setting up a catarrhal condition. Soak the wheatgerm in milk (warm, if preferred) for five minutes before eating. If you prefer, the wheatgerm can be 'short cooked' for two or three minutes in milk. For flavouring or sweetening, use honey only. If this isn't enough for some appetites, the wheatgerm and milk may be followed by fresh or dried apricots and milk or cream. Alternatively a small quantity of grapes. As the condition improves, you can follow the wheatgerm and milk with ripe peaches, or grated apple and milk, or ripe or stewed apricots.
Note: Wheatgerm is not a starch, but a protein.

Mid-morning: Two teaspoons of brewer's yeast powder in a little milk. Alternatively, a thin slice of bread, butter and honey. If, however, you don't take the yeast at mid-morning, it should be taken at four o'clock or before retiring.

Before Lunch: The same vitamins as taken before breakfast, and 1 teaspoonful of olive oil.

Lunch: Two lightly poached eggs—no bread. Followed by grapes, if in season, or papaya. Do not eat bananas at this meal. Bananas are excellent by themselves or with other starch foods, but not with protein (eggs, meat, fish, cheese and nuts are protein).

Before the evening meal: The same vitamins as taken after breakfast with the addition of one pantothenic acid tablet and 1 teaspoonful of olive oil.

Evening meal: A plate of puréed vegetables—such as peas, beans, carrots, parsnips, spinach, pumpkin, cauliflower, etc. Without meat or fish, a plate of steamed vegetables is made more attractive by the addition of cheese sauce or butter sauce. Such a meal may be followed by the mild fruits, such as grapes, peaches, papaya, or banana-cream purée. If one has a juice extractor, carrot, cabbage, or beet-root juice are excellent for ulcers and health. Between meals, sip a glass of milk.

SECOND DAY

Pre-breakfast: Same as before.

Breakfast: Same as before or varied only as suggested.

Lunch: 3oz (85g) cheese with celery. Alternatively, cheese and ripe peaches. Later on, when the ulcer has healed, make cheese and apple your standard luncheon, or a cheese salad.

Evening meal: Poached egg and vegetables—cooked as suggested. By way of a change, about every fourth night, a little grilled fish (but no potato or bread), followed by mild, ripe fruits only (no bananas).

The vitamin dosage, plus the olive oil, remains unchanged.

The Virtue of Potatoes

Dr L. J. Nye has pointed out that stomach ulcer is almost unknown in Ireland and he relates this to the fact that potatoes appear frequently in the Irish dietary. Dr Nye recommends that stomach ulcer patients take two potato meals a day. Potatoes mashed in milk can be taken by themselves as 'mid-meals'. Potatoes contain significant amounts of vitamin C and trace elements. Ulcer patients should ensure that the potatoes they eat are baked or boiled in their skins, as otherwise much of their nutritional value is lost in cooking. Although potatoes are classified as a starchy food, they must not be confused with the factory-processed and refined starches referred to elsewhere in this book, which are of dubious food value.

Coffee, Tea, Smoking and Aspirin

Coffee drinking excites the stomach acids into action when there is no work for them to do. A continual over-stimulation irritates the lining of the stomach and paves the way for stomach ulcers. Tea drinkers are advised to take weak tea with plenty of milk, and no sugar.

Excessive smoking destroys vitamin C in the body and thereby weakens the tissue forming the stomach. According to Dr W. J. McCormick, one cigarette depletes the body of 25mg of vitamin C.

The frequent use of aspirin, in powder or tablet form, is responsible for a good deal of stomach irritation, which can later develop into stomach ulcers. However, this can be reduced by ensuring that vitamin C is taken along with aspirin. For many years it has been known that aspirin causes over-excretion of vitamin C and hence its loss from the body, and may even contribute to its destruction. Vitamin C levels are reduced by chronic ingestion of aspirin as in some arthritic and rheumatic conditions. Now it has been proved in clinical trials that supplementary vitamin C improves the absorption of aspirin; replenishes the vitamin lost by the action of the drug; reduces the irritant action of aspirin on the gastric lining; enhances the pain-relieving properties of aspirin. Other non-steroidal anti-inflammatories used in arthritis have effects similar to those of aspirin. These too are reduced with supplementary vitamin C. It is important that vitamin C is taken at the same time as aspirin and the other drugs to obtain maximum benefit. The usual intake is 50-100mg vitamin C with each aspirin or other tablet.

After the Ulcer Heals

Dr D. T. Quigley advises those who have recovered from stomach ulcers to avoid canned and packaged foods, as they have been robbed of their nutrients by the application of high heat and long storage. He says that such foods are stale and worthless. He forbids his ulcer patients the use of cane sugar, which he calls a slow poison, also white flour products, which between them, constitute over 50 per cent of the food intake of the average person and thereby dilute whatever good, nourishing food the person eats by that amount.

The foods which Dr Quigley allows his patients after their stomach ulcers have healed are meat, milk, raw fruits and vegetables, eggs, unprocessed cheese, wholewheat foods and seafoods. He recommends that the patient consumes a minimum of a pound and half (680g) a day of raw fruits and vegetables, after the complete healing of the ulcer. Any fruit or vegetable that can be served raw, should be eaten raw. Salad vegetables should therefore be preferred to cooked vegetables. From three to six ounces (85-170g) of fresh meat should be eaten daily, cooked as 'rare' as is palatable. No salt meat is permissible, except ham and an occasional breakfast of bacon, and salty foods should be reduced to the minimum.

Dr Quigley says: 'The idea is to reject non-vitamin, non-mineral foods and keep this up for life ... Peptic ulcer is never caused by nervousness, it is associated with it. These persons are irritable and unstable, they are starved generally and specifically.' The reason for this is that 'the nerve disease and the ulcer both go back to a common cause: an over-supply of refined carbohydrates which causes a dangerous reduction of the vitamin and mineral concentration in the blood-stream. Stresses and strains and emotional upsets do not cause ulcer, but merely bring into more prominence conditions which already exist.'

After the ulcer has healed, make sure that you never get another stomach ulcer. You can do this by following Dr Quigley's advice and also by taking every day some brewer's yeast powder (for its vitamin B complex content), some vitamin A and D capsules, vitamin C (250mg) tablets and vitamin E (50mg) tablets or capsules.

Final Words

If any person cares to apply the thirteen curative principles previously recommended, and apply them intelligently and consistently, his stomach troubles should become a thing of the past in a matter of months. Improvement should be certain—except in those long-neglected cases in which the peritoneum has been perforated, or where some incurable ailment has developed. But it requires no small effort of will for the average person to break from his old feeding habits. Habit is so strong that when we change from bad to good feeding habits, the immediate reaction is that we feel the worse for it. But please don't misunderstand this. This phenomenon is simply due to the body reluctantly making its readjustments. Keep to the thirteen curative principles and in a few weeks a great improvement in your general health will make itself felt. The pain after meals should gradually ease and finally disappear. A new feeling of confidence and well-being will permeate body and mind. And, finally, victory over stomach ulcer should follow. But to be rid of a painful disease will not be your only satisfaction. The greater reward will be a far better standard of health and a new zest for life. No small return, you will agree, for the exercise of common sense, a few changes in your eating habits, and a little self-restraint.

Index

JAM

JAMES TOSELAND

The Autobiography

James Toseland
with Ted Macauley

To Mum, Gran and Grandpa,
and big brother Simon
for all the love and support
they've given me.

This paperback edition first published in Great Britain in 2006 by
Virgin Books Ltd
Thames Wharf Studios
Rainville Road
London
W6 9HA

First published in hardback in 2005 by Virgin Books Ltd

A catalogue record for this book is available
from the British Library.

ISBN 0 7535 1103 7
ISBN 978 0 7535 1103 9

Typeset by TW Typesetting, Plymouth, Devon
Printed and bound in Great Britain by
Mackays of Chatham PLC

TED MACAULEY

Ted Macauley is the author of nine books, mostly on motorcycle racing. He was Mike Hailwood's manager and the organiser behind the legendary champion's amazing comeback at the Isle of Man TT in 1978 and then, again, on his winning return a year later.

Macauley was awarded the treasured Seagrave Medal by the Royal Automobile Club for his part in Hailwood's TT fairy-tale comeback after an eleven-year absence from racing on the island's notoriously dangerous and testing track. He was also voted Journalist of the Year.

In between his duties as Chief Sports Feature Writer and Formula One correspondent for the *Daily Mirror*, Macauley wrote three books on his best friend Hailwood – two celebrating his incredible motorbike race career and one as a tribute after Mike's tragic death in a road accident in 1981.

He met James Toseland in 2003 and was immediately impressed by his attitude and his down-to-earth modesty. And still is.

He says: 'It has been an absolute pleasure helping James put together in a book his quite phenomenal and eventful life and career.'

Prologue

ONE VISION

When you cross the line first, wheeling in sheer exhilaration and punching the air in a mixture of relief and regret that the challenge is all over, it is like a reflex expression announcing that, at least for that joyful moment, you are the best.

If I was not a motorcycle racer, I would be the sport's biggest fan. It offers just about every element of excitement possible, from the sheer drama of closely fought battles to as much raw courage on show as you could possibly hope for. It is the thought that you could crash at speed in a charge of bucking, bouncing, sliding machinery which gives the sport a stamp of edgy anticipation. The beauty in close-up of a rider in perfect rhythm, rounding a treacherous bend, and passing a rival or two at the same time, is a joy for both watchers and performers. It is a sport where defining moments threaten your confidence regularly.

Crashing off motorbikes goes with the job. Sometimes it happens when you are not even taking a risk and the bike seems to have a mind of its own. It's not an aspect of the dangerous business that makes you jump for joy, nor does it haunt you every time you race; it's just a fact, a happening – often inevitable. Thankfully, few crashes these days are fatal, but they can still hurt and they can drive you to desperation. And don't I know it. I faced one such serious challenge after a real nasty, career-threatening crash in my first season in British Superbikes.

I had a mega-smash in August 2000 on the Paul Bird Honda, my first really serious spill. I was testing along with a couple of other teams at Cadwell Park ahead of the British Superbike championship when I high-sided for the first time ever, accelerating hard onto the straight. I was hitting 120 mph and feeling good and confident when I suddenly lost control of the bike. It all happened so fast that I didn't have time to react or think about what was happening, or whether it was going to hurt or not, as I cartwheeled into the air. It was my own fault. I lost the rear end and was chucked over the bars, landing on the kerb – just where it was quite sharply edged – and snapped my femur.

The fact that the crash happened so quickly, so violently and without warning, probably saved me from even worse damage. I don't know whether it was the G-forces or what, but I went semi-conscious as I was hurtled head over heels off the pegs and out of the seat. I somersaulted onto the edging, but because I was in a half-blacked-out state, my body was far more relaxed than it would have been if I had anticipated the spill and had tried to cushion it. The worst reaction you can have is to tense up and put your arms and legs down as you plummet towards the ground because that way you are guaranteed to get broken bones. I was so relaxed and mentally out of it that I had no capacity for a reflex self-rescue mission and I hit the floor like a floppy rag doll.

I woke up when my back smacked into tarmac with a sickening impact and heard the noise of the explosive wallop on my spine-protector under my leathers – the juddering jerked me back to my senses. I go cold now when I think of what could have happened if I hadn't been wearing that protector.

I tumbled over a good few times for what seemed an age in an alternating blur of sky and ground. Then I lay dead still because I realised I had hurt my back quite badly and was terrified I might have broken it. A dull, distant ache gradually increased to a lot of pain. I was desperately trying to reassure myself that the situation wasn't that serious – maybe I'd just dislocated a bone or two. Or perhaps I was just waking up from a nightmare. And that's how the shock hits you: you register what has happened, but you refuse to accept it. For those few moments that follow a big trauma like that you are in another world. I kept repeating, 'Oh please, God, just let it be dislocated.'

My right leg had shattered straightaway, with resounding staccato cracks in three places that I can almost hear now. It was wrapped grotesquely and almost impossibly round my neck. The pain was excruciating. But what made the whole awful experience even worse, and more frightening, was that because it was a test day, as opposed to a race event, there was no on-the-spot medical service and I was forced to wait 45 minutes for help to come from outside. In those moments I had to really try my determination to live – it was a nightmare, to say the least.

The situation was reckoned to be so serious and urgent that I was transferred to hospital in an air ambulance helicopter. They said they would not give me too much gas and air in case I passed out, but the way I felt, and the pain I was suffering, I wouldn't have cared. It would have been a blessed relief to be out of it and KO'd. The whole ordeal was upsetting and because I'd had some gas and air that didn't do anything to aid or speed up relief or alleviate the agony, I felt as sick as a dog. A medic jabbed an anaesthetic straight into my arm instead of a vein and missed my bloodstream, so my arm swelled up to about three times its normal size. I was not too well at all and I lost a lot of blood in a six-and-a-half-hour operation. I was told later it was touch and go.

For the first time ever I wasn't worried about racing or the bike, just about myself. I was scared I would never walk properly again. I had screws all over the place, inside my femur (top and bottom), and a sixteen-inch plate to hold the shattered bits of bone together. The surgeon, a brilliant guy, who performed the operation at the Lincoln Hospital, the nearest to Cadwell Park, came to see me and assured me that as the scalpel work and the repair job had gone so perfectly well they had managed not to lose any length on the leg. I would make a full recovery.

I was in bed in hospital for about two weeks and lost a couple of inches of muscle off both thighs. While I was laid up, I got a frame put up around the bed and had a truck tyre inner tube fixed in it so I could fit my feet in and exercise my legs. It was the year Neil Hodgson had his amazing wild-card spree and won both races against all the big, established stars in the World Superbike event at Brands Hatch. There were 100,000 fans – Hodgy's Army – going mad for him. Most of them seemed to be wearing the orange T-shirts of his team's colours – thrown into the crowd or given away by his manager Roger Burnett in a clever bid to drum up fervour for a home favourite. I watched all the action on television from my sickbed, and whatever doubts and fears I'd had about racing again just ebbed away. I was mesmerised – just as surely as I had been in the beginning, long before I found out racing could hurt.

There's no benefit in a glorious Technicolor close-up replay. I try not to watch video replays of my crashes or anybody else's. It's not that the sight of us flying through the air worries me; it's the ouch-factor I don't want to rerun. When you are sitting in front of the television, all black and blue or in plaster with more stitches than a sewing circle, you know what it feels like when racers hit the floor. I wince every time I see it happen and I know the emotions only too well.

I had plenty of time in that hospital room to consider my options: had the crash, and the consequent injuries, done enough to scare me? Would pure bravado keep me fuelled up for racing? Or could I take the perils head-on and try as hard as I could, right on the threshold of survival, knowing now how much it can hurt when things go wrong? This is where people outside any dangerous sport find it difficult to understand how jump jockeys, downhill skiers, Formula One drivers and motorbike racers can't wait to get back into action, even after they have suffered the scariest of near misses and badly damaged themselves doing it. My experience – after several crashes, about nine operations for broken bones, and a lot of time in hospital in great discomfort – is that you return to racing an even stronger competitor than you were before. It has to be that way, or you wouldn't go back at all. Either way, it's a brave decision.

I believe it would make such a massive hole in my life if I stopped racing voluntarily, and not because a crippling injury forced me out. I don't think I could do it. My kicks, the buzz I get from racing and winning, are all in my own hands. I don't want to sit on the sidelines and watch it; I have to be in there, shaping my own fate.

People are always asking me to fully explain how a motorbike racer feels, and whether we get scared, and what it is like to be world champion. Sure, we do get frights because that goes with the territory, but, even after a good few serious spills, breaks and bruises, I am more afraid of failure than injury; I would bet that would be the answer any bike racer would give. The awful frustration you feel when things don't go the way you plan, and the wins stop happening, is far more intense and lasting than any hurt from a crash. That's what makes winning so magical. The pitfalls are so prevalent that when perfection rides with you – when you get every corner just right, your overtaking is smooth and decisive, and your consistency keeps lap times only split seconds apart – the utter triumph of knowing you were spot on lifts you beyond belief. And when you cross the line first, wheeling in sheer exhilaration and punching the air in a mixture of relief and regret that the challenge is all over, it is like a reflex expression announcing that, at least for that joyful moment, you are the best. And it's that feeling that has kept me, and will continue to keep me, in this spot for a long time.

You may have guessed by now that the buzz I get from competition supersedes any slight variance of confidence and cancels out any worries about what will inevitably happen in the next 45 minutes or so, rain or shine, in a committed helter-skelter, full-pelt stampede. I love it. It is my drug. I am hooked. Even the jangling nerves before a race, the adrenalin build-up and the wound-up agitation needed for a vital explosion of energy from the gridline, become enjoyable in a perverse sort of way. When all of this comes together, a wonderful alliance of the elements crucial to success at any sport, the satisfaction is like nothing else in the world.

One

WE WILL ROCK YOU

Freddie Mercury's voice came booming full-volume out of the radio. I twigged that his songs were all about winning and I was instantly a confirmed fan.

After I was born on 5 October 1980, I was taken home to live with my mum and dad in a static caravan in Doncaster. There was Simon, my elder brother by eighteen months, and our golden Labrador, Heidi. With the dog, it made five of us, crammed into our caravan home for about three years. You can imagine what stress my mum must have had to cope with: two babies, a big floppy dog and a husband she was soon to split from. I was only three when Mum and Dad decided to go their separate ways, so I was far too young to realise what had gone wrong. I don't even have pictures in my mind of what Dad looked like. In fact, the only memories I have of that time are of a tin roof over my cot, a plastic Santa Claus and a tatty, broken plastic snowman Mum used to hang on the wall every Christmas.

I have never really been curious about why my dad and mum split up and I don't think I have ever asked. I suppose I always reckoned it was their business and I have learned to live with it. I know for some people they would have to know all the answers, but I can honestly say it never registered as an important thing to worry about. I simply never knew my father and I already had all the love I needed from Mum. We had a special bond because of the closeness you can get in a family where cramped living conditions inspire and teach you to share small comforts. Mum worked hard picking up as much office work as possible, managing a small loans company and bringing home whatever little she could every week. We didn't have a lot of luxuries, but we found that life in the caravan brought us closer together.

After my parents split up, my mother moved us out of the caravan to go and stay with my Grandma Pam and Grandpa Alec in Pontefract. Then we moved with them to Tiverton Park, where I lived most of my life. My grandparents had a home in Wells Road and we bedded down with them until Mum was given a council house in the same village – 8 Waverley Avenue.

Gran had an upright piano in what she called the parlour – the front room and the best, poshest room in the house, usually reserved for special occasions, family visits, etc. The piano was a little brown instrument with a few years on it, but it was still her special treasure, and she loved to play for us, especially at Christmastime. It was just like families and friends must have done in the old days, long before telly and radio. We would all gather round and sing along to her carols. I loved it. I loved the warmth and the close family feeling those times gave me and I was fascinated by the way Gran could do something everybody else was so interested in. She was modest by nature, but when she played the piano and sang, everybody joined in singing the carols and she was in her element. I got to see a different Gran. I guess I enjoyed what I saw as a beautiful change in her so much, that I wanted to copy her. I don't know whether I was an attention-seeker or what, but I was desperate to make everybody else happy just by playing a piano. As soon as I was given the chance to play, I was utterly hooked and became an eager learner. That is how music came into my life.

My brother Simon did not have the slightest interest in playing; he was a total contrast. I could not wait to learn and be as good as Gran; he couldn't be bothered. It was great having an elder brother. Simon had to do all the learning from his mistakes while I was clever me, picking up the pieces, noting where he had gone wrong and making sure I didn't fall into the same traps. We were, and still are, extremely close. We shared a room at home and I must have loved him to put up with the awful smells of his old socks and stuff, which used to come from his end of the bedroom. Or was it the other way round?

At first, Gran's overworked little piano was in great danger from me. I was basically damaging it with my ham-fisted, six-year-old efforts to bang out a tune. She was so lovely and patient with me when I was tunelessly plink-plonking away and trying to unravel the mysteries of the keyboard. I must have had a bit of a gift for it because pretty soon I had learned a few simple little tunes. Then I moved on to tougher stuff and mastered, or probably more accurately, found my way around 'In The Mood', a beaty big dance-band oldie, and then 'The Entertainer'. Suddenly, I was a piano player and Gran was over the moon. Mum, too, was really proud.

Gran realised that there were limits to what she could teach me and that proper lessons from a professional were necessary. I was playing most days and really enjoying it, but I was sceptical, and shy, I suppose, about having lessons because I worried that there would be other, cleverer kids there and they would all be better than I was, making me look daft. I had no idea lessons would be a one-to-one thing. I didn't reveal my fears, not to Gran or Mum, and for a couple of years I stubbornly refused to go to lessons, even though everybody was telling me how good I was and that I would only get better with personal tuition.

Then one day, when Mum was on the loo in the bathroom – she made a lot of critical decisions there – she started calling out to me, really going on at me that I should learn to play properly. I finally relented, but only after I was assured that there would be only me and Pat

Goude, the teacher. There would be nobody sniggering or laughing at me. I couldn't read music, but I did have some simple tunes in my head thanks to Gran, and, armed with them, I made my way up to Mrs Goude's for my first lesson.

Her very nice big house, not exactly The Manor, but massive to a lad from a council terrace, was at the top of the village. I loved lessons from the start. It was the first time I had met a challenge in life – and I was hooked on the excitement. Mrs Goude put me through my limited paces, nodded approval and must have seen something in me that she felt was worth developing. I started going every Monday and Friday after school for my lessons and I can still remember the satisfaction and enjoyment I got. When Gran and Grandpa realised I was dead serious about the lessons, they bought me a second-hand piano to keep and play at home – my absolute pride and joy. Looking back now, it was all a bit *Billy Elliot* – the story of the kid from a Northeast working-class family who wants to be, and becomes against all the odds, a ballet dancer. The difference was that my family were fully behind me. All the way. I guess playing the piano came with a little more street cred, though.

Under Mrs Goude's expert and patient guidance, when I was about eight years old I passed my Grade 1, 2 and 3 piano. I had this vision of going to the London College of Music (now the London College of Music and Media) because I had seen a documentary about it on television. I mentioned my ambitions to my teacher and she said that if I successfully got past Grade 8 I could go to the LCM and, after that, become a professional musician. Well, that was it. There I was, living in a humble little council house with a mum who was struggling to keep a family – and I was already pushing heady dreams. I was way ahead of myself and I certainly had no idea that my own piano would be central to a dramatic and life-altering change in my life.

I was in bed at home one night, half asleep, when I heard somebody playing my piano. I couldn't believe it. I knew my brother hadn't got a note in his head, Mum didn't play, and anyway she had gone out, and it was too late for Gran to be in our house. I wondered who the hell it was. The music I could hear was this great boogie-woogie and rock'n'roll sound, nothing like the stuff Mrs Goude had been playing, and I followed it downstairs and put my head round the door. There was this guy I had never seen in my life playing all these amazing sounds on my piano. I wasn't scared – it was fantastic. All this Ray Charles and Jerry Lee Lewis stuff was echoing around our little living room. It was magic to my ears, and completely different to what I was used to. I was into the classical categories and ragtime. Rock and blues were not on my agenda, but they soon were after I heard more amazing sounds rattle from my upright.

The man had come home with Mum – she introduced him as Ken. Outside, parked on the path, was his Yamaha YZF1000. He was a bike fanatic as well as a superb pianist – talk about a role model – and the difference he made to my life was incredible. Ken was the first person to put me on a bike and show me how to ride. Not only did he introduce me to pop music, he fired me up about motorbikes and he gradually became the father I never knew. He was a biker through and through, an Isle of Man TT race fan and he had done a bit of trials riding – no serious competitions, just riding for the sake of it. The fun of two wheels meant a lot to him and the idea that he could pass on his enthusiasm to two eager kids was a huge appeal.

At junior school I feared I might be considered a bit wimpy. I was tiny and skinny, I had a brace on my teeth, wore glasses – and, horror of horrors to the more macho lads, I was uncool enough to be playing the piano. My nickname was Todo, but some kids sneeringly called me 'The Pianist' – like it was some kind of insult. I wasn't exactly bullied, but I was hardly regarded as a hero to be feared; I certainly didn't look like one. Luckily, if ever I was picked on, I had my big brother, who was renowned for being handy around the playground. Pick on James (never Jim or Jimmy, by the way) and you pick on Simon. The Toseland clan, all two of us, were close. Mess with us at your peril. When Ken came into our lives, it wasn't long before the cruel and dismissive jibes about me playing the piano and looking a bit weird and bookish, gave way to open-mouthed unashamed looks of admiration and awe from the other kids at school. My all-important credit soared. I became a biker . . . a racer.

Ken fascinated me – his motorbike, the way he could play the piano, his genuine interest in me and Simon, and the way he made Mum happy all added up. It was because of him that my life turned so significantly and my future began to take shape. Ken gave me the added security I felt from having a father figure around 24/7. He encouraged me to push myself, take my interests that little bit further and be proud of them. He had all these stories about rock musicians, which I figured was much more interesting than anything the kids at school would say, and I remember hearing him talk about his bike – the language he used made it sound such a powerful and macho thing to do. He was an engineer so it was all 'wheel spin' this and 'cc' that. I was addicted. At eight years of age it was seventh heaven having a man come into my life who had mastered both the two interests I would grow to love, music and bikes, and who was only too happy to treat Simon and me like his own sons. It certainly was not difficult for me to connect with him, especially because when my real dad and mum split up I was too young to remember what must have been a heartbreaking time for my mother. Ken coming along just seemed right and, because Mum was happy, I was happy. Suddenly I was ready to take on the world.

Somehow, I found enough confidence – some people would call it cheek – to ask Mum and Ken if I could have a motorbike. To my absolute amazement, they agreed, and a couple of months later they bought me a second-hand 80 cc trials machine. Simon got one as well because he, too, suddenly found the idea of being a biker incredibly tempting. Ken was unfailingly fair like that – he always had enough time for both of us, and Mum was always keen to not show favouritism. Anyway, there was no way either of us could resist the longing to own a bike – it would make us just about as cool as possible among the other kids at school. I don't know how Ken and Mum afforded the bikes – Mum didn't have any money to spare, but I think Ken had quite a good engineer job and he was a generously spirited guy both with his time and his cash.

After my parents' separation, and just after Ken came on the scene, my dad occasionally used to come and take us out to a park near home, but, to be honest, I never really enjoyed it. This was because we spent most of our time aimlessly hanging about doing nothing except watch the ducks or play on the seesaw and swings. I got bored and agitated very quickly. Dad looked a bit like me – all the Toselands have quite an athletic build and similar face – but that was where the connection between us ended. I don't remember anything about his personality except that I found our time together slightly awkward. He'd turn up because he wanted to spend time with us, but I never ran to greet him. I wanted to be doing the active things that I had grown to love and the result was that Dad and I never really gelled. Simon, who was the spitting image of Dad, got on much better with him than I did. It is something my brother and I have never really talked about, but it did seem that he was more affected by the visits. Awfully, one day he came to pick us up and I threw myself on the floor in a kicking and screaming tantrum because I didn't want to go to the park; I wanted to be playing or riding with Ken. Eventually, it got to the point where we stopped going out with Dad, or he stopped coming for us, and we became increasingly distanced from one another. I was much happier after that. My dad has always been a bit of a stranger and it has always made more sense to me for him to remain so.

Simon and I remained close no matter what. Shortly after Mum and Ken had bought us our bikes we took them to Gran's one Boxing Day for a bit of showing off in her huge back garden at the end of some allotments and Simon ran into the back of me. It was a massive crash and we both fell in a big heap on the ground. I gave him some stick for crashing into me and causing my first accident, but it didn't put me off or scare me and I climbed right back on. From that moment, despite the dangers, my mind was made up that motorcycle racing was what I wanted to do. So I owe my stubborn dedication to biking to Simon, but he was also responsible for the first break of my career. Under Ken's tuition, and with his keenness for us to become competent bikers, we entered trials competitions in the dales around our Yorkshire home. I was in the junior class, which meant that I was faced with having to master obstacles not much more challenging than riding up and over a two-inch-high kerb or over a branch to the finish, and that was that. Being older and having a bigger bike, Simon faced much tougher and more advanced courses, wet routes that demanded more effort than mine, and it put him off – so much so that he stopped. And I stopped, too, just because he had. For a year.

The bikes stayed in the garage and we hardly touched them except for an occasional outing. Instead, while I concentrated on my piano playing, Simon started to think seriously about football. When he was about fourteen he was so good and full of promise that he was invited to join Sheffield Wednesday juniors. All of a sudden, he went from kicking a ball about in the park with his pals on a Sunday afternoon to having to think about maybe one day being a professional footballer. But my brother has never burned with ambition or competitiveness and he missed the *craic* of being with his mates. The close-knit atmosphere he revelled in so much was not there with the Wednesday juniors and he lost any sense of enjoyment of the game. Mum and Ken used to take him to the ground from the other side of Sheffield, a fair trip there and back, and do everything that Wednesday wanted them to do to encourage him to develop his undoubted talent. But he just was not up for it – and he didn't want to carry on. My brother was always destined to be a champion at whatever he did, and that turned out to be being a parent. For my money, he's world champion at that.

In the meantime, my hunger for biking and racing was being reawakened. A lad at school was on about buying a motocrosser and I had been reading all about them in the *Trials and Motocross* magazine. I really fancied one. And you know what it's like when you are at school; if somebody has something, you want it, too. I felt confident I could ride fairly well and handle a bit of extra power, so I asked Ken if I could have a motocrosser. He pointed out, quite rightly and no doubt with increasing and justifiable disappointment, that I had not kept up with my riding on the trials bike that he had bought for me. So he said he would make a deal with me.

'Win a trials championship and I will buy you a motocross bike,' was his promise.

And his ruse worked; I was a fast learner and I couldn't resist a challenge, however high the odds were stacked against me. I took up trials riding again after my year-long lay-off and I did it with renewed vigour. I loved getting up really early, even if it was still dark and cold and often in foul weather, to drive to a windswept and remote trials course somewhere up in the hills, often miles away from my warm bedroom where Simon was still asleep, to slug it out over bone-shaking and wearying mud heaps. Ken would drive us there and he always had taped music blasting out of the car radio. One time he said he was going to introduce me to Queen and I thought he meant Elizabeth and I wondered how he would have managed to get Her Majesty to sing. I had never heard of the band and I had only seen the Queen making her speech at Christmas and didn't fancy the idea of listening to her again. Not at that time in the morning. Then – wham-bang – Freddie

Mercury's voice came booming full volume out of the radio. It was incredible and it sent shivers down my spine. I twigged that his songs were all about winning and I was instantly a confirmed fan. It seemed as if we had a shared motivation – 'We Are The Champions' – and I was inspired to take that uplifting song as my personal anthem. Ken and I used to play it over and over on our way to trials meetings to get ourselves wound up and prepared, especially when it was really cold and uninviting. That was when we felt we needed a booster, a lift to our morale, and Queen and Mercury did it for us.

I missed Simon, and I felt he would have enjoyed the whole atmosphere with Ken and me and Mum and the rousing Queen music and the fun we had. I was only ten, but I was as fired up to be a winner as any older boy with far more experience. I had the added advantage of my mum's unfailing interest and support, and Ken's obvious delight and pride in my good and promising results, never mind wins. He could not have been more of a dad if he had been my real father. It was easy under those conditions to give it my all – or my all as I knew it then. I was just so sorry that Simon wasn't a part of it. He was older than me, with a different set of friends and different interests.

The upshot was that at ten years of age I gave Ken everything that he had asked of me, and more. I won the East Midlands junior championship – and the year after, when I had moved up a grade to C-class, did it again. I was having the time of my young life.

There were people who knew my parallel passion was my piano playing and wondered whether I was worried that I might damage my hands riding trials and motocross, two really tough disciplines that can often carry dangers of injury. Neither Mum nor Ken tried to make me choose between the two pastimes and I honestly never gave the risks a split-second's thought. Anyway, in the heat of competition you never think you are going to get hurt even if you do fall off, and I suppose I had enough childish enthusiasm to believe I'd never crash. It never bothered me and I threw myself into riding as hard as I could while at the same time keeping up with the piano lessons.

I was never torn between the two interests. As much as I loved my music, and as good as I was getting, I was never in any doubt once I was completely certain that I would be a motorcycle rider for ever and ever. It did not trouble me that I was having to split my two hobbies – I loved doing them both, but I found I was getting more fulfilment riding a motorbike than I was playing the piano. Motorbikes, I vowed, would always come first. Then I worked out why: playing music is such a vitally different emotion. According to your mood (glad, sad or indifferent), you can sit down, lift the lid of a piano and, in a world of your own, express, mirror and interpret your innermost feelings through your own hands. If you feel upset, you can slow it down. You can speak with the piano and make it answer back, and that is why it is such a wonderful experience – it reflects your ups and downs, either as a form of escape or a confirmation of your feelings. Anybody who plays will fully understand what I am trying to get at: maybe it is the same if you have mastered the guitar or any other instrument for that matter. I knew that I would always be able to use the piano as a release, but bikes were different. It wasn't an occasional mood that was drawing me towards them – I wanted to, and needed to, be racing all the time. It was a different kind of emotion – more dynamic and important to me.

A teacher at school suggested that as a little diversion I might like to take up the drums, because I had so much aggression in me and sometimes when she was walking past the room where I was playing she thought I must have been dismantling the place. I have not a clue where my attitude came from or where the teacher got that idea. I did not, and still don't, have a temper – that is a blessing in a cruel cut-and-thrust sport like mine. But what I did have, and still do, is this need to release pent-up energy. That is why motorcycles have always played such a crucial part in my life; right from the first time I climbed on one and fired it up.

At high school I had plenty of aggression and I was cheeky, but with enough of a smile to get me out of trouble. It always seemed to me they were trying to teach me stuff in music lessons that I already knew or could not be bothered to learn and take in – playing the block and triangle, for example. That bored me stiff. They had a drum kit in music lessons, too, and of course that's what all the kids wanted to play. Not me. It was the piano or nothing. So when they gave me a go on the drums I used to bash them like hell, enjoying the racket and sense of release, but never giving a thought to any notion of learning how to play them properly. Anyway, I could get all the noise and tension out of my system with my bike.

I didn't think schooling was important because I was never in any doubt that I would be either a racing motorcyclist or a professional pianist just as soon as I could get out into the grown-ups' world. Everything else was second best and it affected my concentration in the classroom. I was out to have a good time racing and, while I noticed them, girls were not part of that. No way. They would have been regarded by me as a nuisance. In any case, I was painfully shy. I just wanted to be on the fringe, only pushing myself when it came to racing. Girls were background creatures in my life. How things change ... As far as school went academically I was fine, not brilliant, but OK if a subject grabbed me. I only struggled at business studies. That was because the woman teacher, I suppose in her twenties, was really nice-looking and I couldn't concentrate on anything but her.

It is embarrassing now when I think back to those days, especially when I seemed to be going through one of those spells of awkwardness that can make adolescents little horrors. I used to embarrass my mum about lots of things. Like, if we went to somebody's house or people came to our place and I was cold, I would sit right up by the fire and some well-meaning person would kindly ask if I was all right. Instead of being polite and tactfully saying I was OK, I would blurt out that, no, I wasn't, I was bloody freezing. Mum always tried to instil in me the need to be polite. It was the way she was brought up and it was the way she wanted me to be. Trouble was, I didn't know the meaning of the word or understand the subtleties of manners and acceptable behaviour and, even though it was not my intention to be rude or ungrateful or offend anybody for their concerns, I would say straightaway what was in my head. Whatever way it came out. Good or bad. But mostly awful. And to Mum's complete embarrassment.

I could not wait to leave school. All my classmates were planning their day jobs – being a pilot, joining the army, being a footballer – and I had no such thoughts. It was a bit daft and short-sighted really because if I had crashed, hurt myself badly enough never to race again, or damaged my hands so that I could not play the piano, I would not have been able to do anything that had driven me forwards to my dreams. And, of course, that is all they could be before I would be old enough to make it a living. Just a dream.

I remember going to visit a careers officer in my first or second year and him asking me what I wanted to do. I told him I was going to be a bike racer, simple as that. He said, 'Come on, now, you can't do that. You need a trade.' My brother was training to be a joiner so I thought maybe I could just say that I'd like to do a trade to keep him happy. He started looking through his files for something suitable and said, 'Would you prefer to work weekends?'

I remember thinking: I only want to work weekends. Friday practice, Saturday qualifying and I'll be home by Sunday. I don't think he was very impressed.

There was one other setback I had to overcome before I could really get down to serious racing. The need to be

23

ultra-fit is crucial. That goes without saying, because the physical demands at the speeds you have to go and the heaving and yanking of the bike into and out of corners and throughout overtaking, as well as the G-forces that jumble up your innards in acceleration and braking, can mean the difference in a split second of sudden weakness or frailty between soaring success or abject failure. I have always had a love for sport. Both my dad and mum were trim and slim and I inherited the build with pretty good muscle tone: in fact, just about everybody in the Toseland family is on the acceptably lean side of skinny and the genes that came down the family line left me, naturally, quite athletic. I certainly did not have to work at getting myself into the right shape, say, for cross-country, a favourite sport of mine, or tennis or any of the outdoor games I really do enjoy. Not like a lot of my mates at school, who used to hide in the hedgerows, and maybe have a smoke, wait until the honest runners like me returned sweating and aching from the country, then dodge out again from under cover and jog fresh as a daisy to the finish line.

However, looming inside me was a problem I'd had without knowing since I was a toddler: concave ribs. Basically, the left-hand side of my ribcage went in instead of out and it got to the stage where they were bending a little too close to my lungs. The dangers inherent in that are obvious. It was not giving me any desperate problems or anxious moments – but I must have suspected or noticed something unusual because when I was about fourteen it suddenly became more noticeable and I told my mum it didn't feel quite normal. She took me to the hospital right away and an X-ray proved me right. A surgeon said I needed an operation as soon as possible. It was a massive cutting job and, to this day, I have a vivid scar down my chest to remind me. If my ribs had been allowed to carry on growing, developing with me, they could have started to dig in and stab me, affecting my lungs and my breathing and perhaps, the doctor said without explaining what exactly, could cause other problems. Earlier rather than later was his advice on the operation. And I was really poorly afterwards for about six months. I thought I was normal, fit and healthy. It just goes to show that you can never be one hundred per cent sure, and if you have the slightest suspicion something is amiss you have to be sensible and get it looked at and fixed, because it won't go away on its own. In my case, it was timely because it eliminated any problems that could have developed later on in life.

It wasn't feasible to think so then, but when I look back at the obstacles that could have undermined my ambitions to be a racer, it was like they were all being wiped out one by one by some greater good. In the future I would have more demanding and completely unexpected situations to contend with, but for now, I was just at the time in my life when things could not have been more exciting – I was awakened to the magic of road racing.

CONTENTS

ACKNOWLEDGEMENTS

Thanks to Ken, Kirsty, Bailey and Jack, Grandma and Granddad Toseland, Uncle Michael and Aunt Sue, Eric and Sue Grayson, and John and Kathleen Jones.

To everyone at Honda and Ducati for giving the bike to support my dream, and to Roger Burnett whose friendship and experience guided me along the way.

To all my friends from Kiveton Park and my fans who have stuck with me through the good times and bad.

And to all at Virgin Books for giving me the opportunity to talk about my life.

Two

BICYCLE RACE

I would try to escape by jumping on the motocross bike and riding off hell for leather as fast and as crazily as I could. On my own I went back to the disused colliery top where I used to ride and climbed as high as I could, wanting, I suppose, to get as far away from thing as possible. Then I sat astride the bike, arms stretched towards the heavens, and just screamed.

The operation I had on my ribs left me feeling weak and unwell and with hardly any energy for a while, but it could not dampen any enthusiasm or ambition I had for being a racer. I was only thirteen when, after a year as a newcomer in motocross, I had to be moved up to the 125 cc class. However, for the group, I was really short. My feet could not reach the ground and I never felt in control when I was riding the bike. Instead, the bike was riding me, and my confidence suffered. It put me off. The bike was just too big for me and, just when I had been doing well in trials and winning things, I was finishing nowhere in motocross. The frustration was enormous, but there was nothing I could do about my little legs to enable me to ride the bike properly.

Road and short-circuit racing, despite Ken's keenness on it, had never grabbed me at all. However, I started watching Grand Prix on television when the likes of Wayne Gardner, Kevin Schwantz and Mick Doohan, all world 500 cc champions, were in their spectacular pomp and turning in thrillers every time they raced. I noticed you did not need height to be a road racer. To be jockey-sized like me, provided you were strong enough, was OK. So I asked Ken if we could swap the motocrosser for a road bike and go racing. He was, as usual, fully behind me and we (well, he) bought an ageing TZR125.

It had a few modifications, but it was still a bit too big for me. We used to take it to a nearby industrial estate car park to give it a whirl, but we never raced it – I was just fourteen, and was too young. For a year I messed around on it in private, but I knew by the way the bike felt under me, the power it had, the way it handled and the buzz it gave me, that I had found the sport for me. I had loved trials and enjoyed the competition, but I didn't get as much of a kick out of motocross because I was only OK at it. Perhaps that was because I had only given it one year and had been put off by having to move up to the 125 cc class – that and the fact I could not properly handle the machine. Now I had spent a year getting used to a road-racing machine it was time to move on and get stuck into some competition so that I could see how I could measure myself against other lads.

We targeted a series being organised by the Junior Road Racing Association. It was a British Championship, but a locally run event with no trophy at the end of it, staged at tracks all over the country. We bought an 80 cc Cagiva from Kenny Tibble, a good novice racer, who had won the series the year before. And, as I had no road-racing gear at all, as part of the deal we bought his leathers, which were far too big for me. I also wore a bright-blue helmet that belonged to an auntie and was given to me by my uncle. The baggy leathers were red and white and very second-hand, so you can imagine I cut quite a colourful and pathetic figure, with a lot to live up to kitted out like that. Even the knee-sliders were out of position, halfway up my leg and poking out – nowhere near the setting they should have been to be of any use when I got my knee down painfully in the corners.

My first real race was at Cadwell Park, in Lincolnshire, on the short circuit. I had been there with Ken as a spectator when I was building up my change in biking ambitions and had been really fired up watching the professionals hard at it on a tricky track.

We had a Vauxhall Cavalier with a trailer to carry the bike. Mum didn't come so it was just Ken and me. At the circuit there was a cousin of mine who raced with Ken's brother-in-law and another lad, Stephen, who had a caravan. We only had a car and an open trailer with nowhere to relax, so we blagged coffee and tea from everybody else's hospitality areas and used anybody's caravan we could to get out of the weather.

Tough going as it was, it was tremendous fun. The atmosphere in the paddock was unbelievably friendly; everybody helped everybody else whether they knew each other or not. If somebody wanted to borrow some tools or a tyre or some oil or anything, even if they were going to be racing hard against each other in half an hour's time, everybody mucked in and helped. It was my first introduction to the comradeship that bikers at all levels seem to share. Self-interest, with no favours offered or wanted, is kept strictly to the track. You would not expect it to be any different among a fiercely committed bunch of racers all riding as hard as they could to win, but off track it was just like Ken had said it would be. The warmth of friendship was everywhere, everybody threw out a welcome and newcomers such as me were especially greeted and made to feel at home.

By now Ken and I were getting even closer. He and Mum had become engaged. She wore his ring, but I don't recall any talk of marriage – at least not in front of me. It was clear they were a serious item. Ken even talked about changing my name from Toseland to his, Wright. I found that I needed Ken's company and counsel to keep me calm before a race. I used to get butterflies and be nervous on the way to the meeting and I never liked being in a group of lads, unlike other guys who find it a good way to relax. I much preferred to take myself off and be alone somewhere, however genuinely pally people in the paddock wanted to be. I have always been a watcher, an onlooker, never part of a gang or group. At tracks, right up to today, I have always opted to stand back and take in the scene, watch the other guys, study them and what they do and how they handle the build-up to the race. It is part of my preparation and has become second nature to me now – though I bet a good few people must believe I am either really stuck up or scared to death. It is neither, far from it; it is just my way of dealing with the tension and making sure I get the last vestige of advantage from watching the riders on the grid.

When I sit on the bike, I am so concentrated, so channelled to the job and the explosion of power and the hustle and bustle of the stampede of a start that I cannot later recall any of the emotions or feelings or doubts I may have had. It is all a blur. At fourteen I was the same, even in my first race. Most of the lads were a year older than I was, and there were about fifteen of us ready to go. Grid placings were decided by us each pulling a numbered peg out of a hat. Not that it made too much difference to me. I was a lousy starter, so it didn't make any odds to me where I was. Front, back or halfway along, I always struggled to get away and had to make up for a sluggish start with a determined ride.

That first early-season race in a cold March of 1995, freezing to death in those red and white leathers, was a two-leg event and I managed a couple of fourth places. You can imagine how chuffed I was – just off the podium in my first road race. I could not wait to get home to tell Mum all about it. And Queen was with us all the way. I felt like a champion. I knew I had found what I most wanted to do. Not that the notion of being a full-time road racer thrilled my mum too much. She did not mind the trials or even the motocrossing because they were not anywhere near as dangerous, but she did not approve of my new career plan too much. And why should she? She had a son who had become so proficient at the piano that he was going to go to the London College of Music. She was a concerned mum and wondered what the hell I was doing arsing about on a motorcycle with the ever-present threat of coming home with a broken this or that, when I could just play the piano and join the London Symphony Orchestra, with no greater danger to my health and wellbeing than the piano lid falling on my fingers.

Then, just to underpin her worst fears, I had my first crash. It was at Darley Moor in my third race. I high-sided my little 80 cc Cagiva at the hairpin and that, believe me, was something of an achievement. The bike was lucky to make 12 bhp – lawnmowers spin up better. However, it did make it and over the top it flicked me, so I landed on my head with a mighty bang.

The hurt was nothing compared to the embarrassment. It was the first time I had taken a tumble on tarmac and it took the wind out of me. The leathers did not have much padding, so you can imagine that when I landed in a big untidy heap on the black stuff, I felt it. I limped rather red-faced across the track and sat on a tyre wall, realising for the first time that road-race bikes can, and do, bite back when you least expect it. I spent the waiting time making up an excuse: when I got back to the paddock, I moaned that there was some oil on the track. I don't imagine that for one second anybody believed me, but nobody criticised or blamed me.

I probably did not realise it at the time, but I had been building up confidence and was getting better and better, even beginning to think that racing was quite easy. I'd had those two fourths first time out and in the next round I got a couple of second places. So when it came to the Darley Moor meeting, I was more than likely a bit too bold for my own good when going around the hairpin. Clearly, the bike didn't like it. High-siding, that most fearsome of spills, is always likely to be nasty. OK, you do get used to falling off and rolling with it, but when the bike digs in all at once and hurtles you out of the saddle it flicks you really high. High enough to give you the time to realise that when you come down again it is certain to hurt. Luckily, I did not break anything, not even a finger, until 1998, eight years after I had begun racing. And that's quite rare.

Sometimes I wonder where I would be in life if I hadn't had Ken's guidance while I was growing up. I don't want to sound off like a preacher, but I am convinced that a fair proportion of young people who break the law would not be doing it if they had had well-intended influences and support in their lives. We all need positive aims and if only someone could give them the help they need to build themselves a future, maybe they'd have a better shot at things. Without crucial direction or anybody able or willing to steer you, you can easily nosedive to nowhere, and with all those unpredictable hormones messing up your mental balance as a teenager, it can land you in big trouble.

Central to my safe passage into the adult world were the values and patience that came to me through Ken. It would be impossible and unfair of me to understate the influence he brought to bear on my childhood and the untiring encouragement and devotion he gave me. Maybe he saw in me what he would have most liked to have been: a racer, and a winner.

From my side, I was the most willing of pupils, eager both to please him and Mum, and find satisfaction and pride in my own skill. It's a dedication I found easy to follow, and always have done. Then again, you usually do *if* you are getting the quality and depth of love you need to boost you towards your goals. I think that goes for most challenges in life, whether you want to be a champion sportsman or a success at business; it's just as they say, encouragement is the lifeblood of achievement. Whatever doubts invade your confidence, they can be alleviated by the closeness of somebody whose opinion you respect. That, in my case, was Ken, my father figure.

I was lucky. Whatever aggressive instincts burned inside me, and believe me there were plenty, they found an outlet, a safety valve, in my all-embracing enthusiasm for playing the piano and riding a motorbike right to the edge. I was doubly lucky that I had a mum and a man who backed me to the hilt, leaving no room for self-doubt. There was far more for me in the thrill and excitement of competition, both with the piano and the bike, that kept me off the street corners and out of the sort of trouble that seemed to lure too many lads of my age and background.

Mum and Ken used to have arguments, big ones at times, and she would rage out of the house, slam the front door almost off its hinges and storm off in her car. A little while later, I would hear the door go again and Ken would drive away to go and look for her. Sometimes I used to lie in bed at night listening to their fights, being desperately unhappy about the rows and worrying if the tensions would split them up. Then the doors would be slammed twice and two cars would be driven off into the night. Simon and I would both be awake, but not saying anything to each other, not letting on that we could overhear the arguments that were so loud and prolonged that it was impossible to sleep. The rows became almost the norm, as close as Mum and Ken obviously were, but my brother and I never mentioned it. It never got physical, Ken was not that sort of bloke. He would never hit Mum. However, the shouting was violent; I used to put a pillow over my head to shut out both the noise of the yelling and the hurt the rows caused me to suffer. The rows weren't about anything in particular – they just seemed like everyday stuff that people tend to argue about, but I admit now I was a little biased on Ken's side because of the dad-and-lad closeness of the relationship we had built up. That did not mean I loved my mum any the less, but my biking, and the meetings, made me close to Ken. I won the Junior Road Racing championship in 1995 under his guidance and was about to begin another title series. Simon was more on Mum's side because he was at home more than I was. When Simon changed his plans to be a pro-footballer with Sheffield Wednesday, he no longer had training, and was spending more time hanging around with his pals or at home while I concentrated on the racing.

Luckily, whatever awful atmosphere was created by the frequent fall-outs, it was softened by visits to my grandparents. They had a blissful, fairy-tale marriage, so in their company I knew what a warm and loving relationship could be like. Every day after school I went to their house to have tea and play Gran's piano. I reckon now, without realising it at the time, that the reason I looked forward to going to my gran and grandpa's home so much was because it was calm and peaceful. There were never any arguments and if they ever did have words, never serious rows, she would just flick him with a tea towel and that was an end to the matter. It was old-fashioned, it was lovely and it was comforting. Even though Ken was my father figure right from the beginning, Grandpa was my mentor, a really strong character who I could turn to if ever I needed any advice or help, say, with homework. Nothing was too much trouble for him. Really, I was blessed being surrounded by such caring people, ring-fenced, I guess, from the harsher realities of the world.

The split-ups and noisy walkouts between Mum and Ken became more frequent, even though they made big efforts to mend the damage. I was too young to work out the complexities, and I guess I never will. I just fretted that my biking might be affected if Ken opted out altogether. I figured that if they had no relationship, there would be no motorbiking, so that meant I always wanted them to get back together.

I remember going to Gran's house after school and finding Mum in bed in their spare room. She was in a mess, an absolutely terrible mess, confused and a nervous wreck. She didn't know what to do with herself. And that's when it clicked with me and I thought: Hang on, this is my mum – she shouldn't be in this state over a relationship for whatever reason; it's not good for her. The damage on all sides was deepening and I could see now that Mum was beginning to get ill with stress and depression.

For once, I did not go out riding with Ken and leave Mum with Simon. I wanted to be close to her as well as my brother who was always by her side. Ken knew he was a massive pull to me because of the racing. I resisted the offer for once and said I was sticking with my mum. I cannot explain just how difficult a decision that was for me to take, particularly because I was really getting the hang of the sport. I began to realise, too, that Mum only went back to him after a split because of the part he played in my biking ambitions.

I used to practise on my motocross bike at an old, closed-down quarry not far from home, and Ken, of course, knew it and where I would be on any given day. He came to see me to try and persuade me to go racing with him even though he was officially separated from Mum. Even though I feared my racing would be at a risk if I turned him down, I took one of the boldest decisions of my young life and said no. Ken had also bought my brother a Vauxhall Nova because Simon was taking driving lessons. I don't know for certain, but I suspect it was a bit of a crafty trick to get our kid on his side to help him get back together again with Mum. However, she had deteriorated to a state so serious it was worrying enough for me to put aside my own interests and be concerned instead about her welfare, even if that meant I had to pack the racing in.

We moved house from 8 Waverley Avenue to 39 Stoney Bank Drive, a newly built estate not far away. It was supposed to be a break for the good, but it's funny how you look back on your decisions now. One day we went out and left Simon's car parked in our garage at Stoney Bank Drive. It was the postlady who heard the engine running in the closed-up garage and saw there was smoke pouring from under the doors, so she reported her find to the police who made the discovery. Ken had killed himself. He gassed himself with exhaust fumes from Simon's car in our garage.

Ken was clearly broken by the sure-fire certainty that Mum was never going to be with him again. Their relationship had gone way beyond the acceptable and it could not continue on its destructive path causing my mum such mental and emotional anguish. I reckon he knew that it was all over and that the woman who had become the love of his life had had enough pain. I understand he had an extra-special affection for me, too, but the arguments between them had reached a stage where it was all too much for my mum to bear. The heartache was not worth it and I firmly believe that if they had carried on seeing each other she would not have been here now. Not that she would have done anything silly like harming herself, but she would have made herself so poorly she could well have died.

I was at my gran's with all the family when the police came and told my mum what had happened and that Ken was dead. When she told me, I felt that my world had shattered. I was riddled with guilt because I always felt I was his trump card, the vital key to him getting back together with Mum. It was always me that stopped with him through the good and the bad times because it suited me and my aims, and, anyway, I liked him and revelled in his company. It was always through, and because of, me and his backing for my biking that Mum went back to him. But when he had clearly reached his lowest ebb and was feeling the worst, with the bleak prospect of never getting back the relationship he valued so much, I had deserted him to be with Mum. I had turned him down when he asked me to go racing. It was probably the final straw.

There is, naturally, a feeling of guilt when something this tragic happens. I was so angry, really raging, and I came close to giving up the bikes. With the rage rushing around inside me, I needed to offload – my energy levels were at flood level. It was building up to the stage where I couldn't grieve properly. I didn't understand. I wanted to cry, but there was no real outlet for the amount of pain I felt – my world was just crumbling under my feet.

Mum later told me, when I was old enough to understand, that Ken was a schizophrenic. He had a personality disorder and mood swings that were mystifyingly unfathomable. I never picked up on it at the time, being so young, but it did explain why those rows could reach such dramatic levels. When he and Mum argued his whole attitude swerved away from normal – but when he was nice, he really was just that. In the full fury of a mood swing, which would come on ever so quickly, his words were harsh and horrible. My friends all told me their mums and dads argued, so I never thought Mum's regular rows with Ken were abnormal. I accepted the fights as being just how things are among grown-ups. Looking back, they did throw some truly hurtful slurs at one another.

I was bitterly angry with God for taking Ken. I was furious at Ken for killing himself; a coward's way out, I thought. I wanted to hit back and I was fired up to a degree that could have been dangerous. I got myself out of it by making sure I kept myself busy. At first, when the ire was at its fiercest and the frustration I felt was almost overpowering, I would try to escape by jumping on the motocross bike and riding off hell for leather as fast and as crazily as I could. On my own I went back to the disused colliery top where I used to ride over the old slag heaps on my motocrosser and climbed as high as I could, wanting, I suppose, to get as far away from things as possible. Then I sat astride the bike, arms stretched towards the heavens, and just screamed.

I ached to cause trouble, but didn't have the conviction to really rebel because of all the control and clear thinking Ken had so wisely urged me to have in my racing. It was a disciplined attitude that overflowed into my life and left me without the necessary wildness or abandon to follow through as a bad boy. Still, I wanted to push the limits and I just rode around aggressively and fast, right on the edge. Then I'd go back to the warm and relaxing tranquillity of my gran's house. She and my grandpa understood what I didn't understand myself: my need to release my rage and pay a dutiful homage to my own sorrow. I'd put the bike away until the next time I felt I was being crowded by the utter sadness of it all. That waste of a life and the loss of the helpmate I felt had abandoned and cheated me were turning my emotions inside out. I have never revealed before now how deeply disappointed and robbed I felt. It was a defining episode, a highly personal and life-forming experience, which I have kept as my secret down the years.

My manager, Roger Burnett, calls me the Secret Squirrel. I suppose he is right. I do not let too much of me show if I can help it. Unlike the way my grandparents showed their love, Simon, Mum and I have never been an affectionate touchy-feely sort of family, not demonstrative in any way. It wasn't a surprise that Mum kept her emotions locked up inside. I cannot recall her ever being in tears around me – not even when Ken committed suicide in our home. But she was ill. Her depression was so serious I don't think she was in her right mind at the time. Under normal circumstances you would react, I am sure, to such a trauma with floods of unashamed tears. I don't think she had the capability to respond as other women might have done when they had just lost someone they had loved for about ten years.

The pain, however, did not stop there. Six months later my beloved Grandpa – Alec Billam, really called Albert, but he hated the name – died and, once more, Mum was left picking up the pieces and striving to make sense of the unbelievable feelings all around her. Seeing her lose her father to a heart attack, ten years after he'd had a quadruple bypass, meant even more heartbreak. All the time I was unwittingly getting stronger, being forced to cope with the severest setbacks imaginable – good grounding for my future. I was only fifteen.

Grandpa was the only other member of the family who was competitive: he flew racing pigeons. He and my Uncle Michael, Mum's brother, used to go off to competitions together. When Grandpa came to watch me race, Michael resented that because he, just like me, wanted Grandpa with him. That's how popular he was with everybody.

Seeing Mum was like extra coal being thrown onto the fire inside me after Ken's suicide and Grandpa's death. Me, Simon and Gran had to be positive. My gran was wonderfully strong after Grandpa had gone. He was all she had, she loved him to bits, and to lose him when he was just 58 must have devastated her. She is such a resilient lady that we never saw her in tears despite her heartbreak – she would not want to compromise anybody else's emotions. I had never seen anybody grieve without showing it. I knew her so well that I could see straight through her and it was pitifully painful to watch her suffer, but be too proud to allow anybody else to share her sorrow. She would have hated to be a bother.

My bond with Mum was getting stronger all the time. As young as I was, I could work out that her hurt and her losses were destroying her and I instinctively wanted to be there for her and lessen the pain as best a fifteen-year-old could. I was scared she was crumbling to bits. Dreams to be a full-time racer were shoved right to the back of my mind because I was being overtaken by other, more pressing, family priorities. The motocrosser in the garage was a device to let off steam; being a professional was not at the top of my thoughts, it wasn't the be-all and end-all and I didn't think it was what I was going to do for a living.

My piano playing, too, became a useful means of masking my own concerns and losing myself. I am not an emotional sort of guy. I have rarely found time for tears because it takes a lot to upset me, but like I did then, I can unburden myself of the threat of upset or breakdown by playing and, in a way special to me, let the piano talk me out of my bad mood and into a better one. Whether it is to fend off tension or tears, it is unique and, at times, quite beautifully satisfying.

I am fortunate enough to have always had my racing to let my frustration burn out on the track. Luckily, I opted to carry on despite the setbacks that floored me psychologically for a while. If I had not, Lord knows what might have happened to me. I think I might well have gone off the rails. Mercifully, all those ingredients of self-control and self-motivation that I mentioned earlier remained deeply instilled in me long after Ken had gone.

Up to all the arguments and the problems between Mum and Ken, and then the bereavements, particularly Grandpa's death because I loved him so much, I had had such a normal and simple life, doing everything I most wanted to do. The events I had to cope with, without realising it at the time, certainly did help form my character and I found inside myself a strength that could convert setbacks into positive energy. I do wonder if I would be quite as strong on a motorbike as I am now if I had not experienced all those early dramas that swamped me as a young boy.

Today, I recognise in myself calmness and an ability to cope with difficulty that I firmly believe I would not have if I had not been confronted by so many traumas as a lad, finding his feet in life. Certainly, the tremendous pressures of racing, the severe demands of professionalism and the money that goes into it, do not seem to me to be the big deal or worry they are to other guys in the sport. I just do not lose my bottle.

Three

BREAKTHRU

Suddenly, here's me, sixteen years old and all excited, marching into the kitchen saying, 'Mum, I've met this guy up at the pit and he said he will set me up racing. I only need ten thousand pounds.'

Just like I was asking for a tenner.

She nearly had a seizure.

There have been more ups and downs, twists and turns and character-testing moments in my life than any presented on the 37¾ miles of the Isle of Man TT course – for me, the world's most challengingly treacherous track. Life, it seemed to me as a teenager, just kept on unfairly throwing upset and disappointment in my face. I couldn't keep track of the incidents that crept up on me to test my resolve. But with every challenge, I gave my increasingly worried mum even more assurance that I wanted to be a racer.

I tried to console Mum over the losses of Grandpa and Ken, as well as any young innocent boy could, and slowly but surely the desire to go racing came back to me. I don't suppose I had sense enough to understand that her fears were shaped by the dangers of motorcycle racing.

Just as things were settling down, a cousin of mine who she was very close to, was killed racing a 125 cc at Cadwell Park. He was only 26. That just about put paid to any sympathy she had for my pestering her to buy me a half-decent bike. However, sad though I was at his being killed, it failed to put me off or scare me from racing and I would not let go. He was a lunatic on public roads, so his mum and dad reasoned the best and safest way for him to get the wildness out of his system was to let him go racing. I insisted that his death had not altered my feelings and, even though I was still at high school, one way or another I was going through with it and would somehow find the money to fund my aims.

Mum could see my determination was unshakeable and gradually came round to my way of thinking: I think I just wore her down. I must have been like a torturer, but I didn't feel guilty. My dream was far stronger than it has ever been. Since stopping road racing to be with my mum as often as I could to help her recover from her grief, I missed biking badly, and the passion to get back to it as soon as I could was unquenchable.

We just had to move away from the house where Ken had committed suicide – there was too much sadness connected with it and we could not bear to live there any longer – so we flitted to the other end of the village into a semi-detached house. There was a bit of money left over from the sale of our house in Stoney Bank Drive and somehow, don't ask me how, Mum had scraped some savings together to keep us all going.

I still used to try and get my kicks and find a vent for my energy on my motocrosser over at the old colliery, up and over the slag heap, or just hurtling around the muck and grime and coal dust of the derelict and deserted pithead. It used to get boring at times because I was usually there on my own. Sometimes, if I heard another bike in the distance I would ride over to see if it was somebody I could have a race with, a bit of playtime, because I missed the competition so much.

One day I could hear somebody giving a bike some serious stick so I belted over and found a guy on a 250, absolutely flying at breakneck pace, very impressively, in a figure of eight around a bunch of trees. I joined in, so we were hurtling around, with me trying my hardest to keep up. He was pretty handy, bloody quick and full of confidence. After a while he stopped and when I rode over to him he took his helmet off. I didn't recognise him even though, as I found out later, he lived in the same village as me. He introduced himself. His name was Mick Corrigan and he had finished second for Yamaha in the British championship. No wonder he was too quick for me!

We had a bit of a chat. He asked me who I was, where I came from, how did I manage to be so handy a rider at such a young age and why I was so regularly at the colliery. He told me he was switching to Honda for the championships in '97, so he was obviously pretty well tied up and busy with his title chasing. However, something must have impressed him about my riding. I don't know how, but he managed to find my telephone number and gave me a call with an offer to race a bike he could get his hands on – a brand new CB500 Honda. I nearly jumped down the phone. Can you imagine my excitement? Here was this real road racer, one of the best in the country, asking me if I wanted go racing. Did I?! It was January and I was at home doing nothing except school and studying for my GCSEs. I didn't hesitate: 'yeah, yeah, yeah' came tumbling out of my mouth without a split-second's thought.

'But it'll cost some money,' he warned.

'I'll talk to my mum,' I said, 'I'm sure it'll be all right. I'll call you back.'

Mum was still struggling financially and, even with her small loans business, she was striving to make ends meet. And, suddenly, here's me, sixteen years old and all excited, marching into the kitchen saying, 'Mum, I've met this guy up at the pit and he said he will set me up racing. I only need ten thousand pounds.' Just like I was asking for a tenner.

She nearly had a seizure.

'Ten thousand pounds! You must be kidding.'

I was so excited that I had been offered a brilliant ride that I lost sight of the amount. Then Mick rang back and said, 'Sorry, I miscalculated – it's fifteen grand.' And that brought a firm 'no' from Mum.

'I just can't do it,' she said. 'Impossible . . . impossible.'

However, I was adamant and persistent to the point of what must have been relentless mental torture, and finally she agreed, after very many long-drawn-out conversations, to find the outlay. How she did it, I can't imagine. She stipulated that this was a one-off, a one-and-only chance. And she insisted that she was going to have to give Simon some money, too, because it would not be fair to him if she forked out just for my benefit. She was always scrupulously fair-minded: what was good for one son had to be matched in kind with the other one. It worked both ways. Simon was never jealous and there was never any animosity between us. Just because I had an expensive hobby (two, in fact, with my piano playing) Mum usually spent more money on me than on my brother, but he never griped or accused her of preference. Anyway, the upshot was that, without even knowing Mick, she funded the restart of my road racing.

Mick was a loveable rogue, renowned as a hard man in the paddock and a guy you did not mess with. He set about doing a superb job in getting me into good shape for the sport I most wanted to do. He had broken a collarbone and had had to miss the first part of his British championship, which meant he could give a bit more time to me, getting me right for the upcoming season. I had a few outings on his 600 Honda and got fitter and fitter. All at once, like some long overdue blessing after all the recent heartbreak and upsets, events started to go right. Things were working out for me.

We did not have any sponsorship and I hadn't a clue how to work on the maintenance of my bike. I was a technical dunce. I couldn't drive, either, and in any case I was too young to hold a licence, so we had to work hard to find somebody to take me. To be frank, I don't think Mick believed I would be up to much or have any chance, so he didn't take me to Brands Hatch. I went with his brother Bob and the mechanic, Dane, instead.

Mick was in for a mega-surprise. It must have shocked him later when we phoned him and told him I had qualified two and a half seconds faster than the second-placed lad in the Newcomers' Class.

From a chance meeting with Mick Corrigan one day at a deserted and dirty pithead, here I was at Brands Hatch, the famous championship circuit near London with its fantastic history and reputation, and where the likes of world motorcycle champions John Surtees, Mike Hailwood and Barry Sheene, among many other legends, had made their mark. That was like ... wow! I still can't get my head around how overwhelming it is.

I was so quick that they wanted me to be upgraded to the National race, but there was an age restriction and I was too young at sixteen, so the organisers ruled I wasn't allowed to take part. It caused a big row with the officials, and Mick, who had been told by Bob that I was barred, was so furious that he came down on Friday night to dig his heels in and get me into the National event. He argued that I was fast, I would be lapping the other guys inside two laps and I should get a rightful place on the grid. I was so naive and inexperienced that I just got on the bike and rode the wheels off it without any real race craft or knowing what the hell I was doing. I did what came easily and naturally to me and went for it as hard as I could. I had no idea who the other riders were that I was up against. To me, whatever their reputations, they were there to be beaten, they were in my way. I know there were people who could not believe that this unknown upstart kid from the sticks, the rawest of rookies at this level, could be so fast. I just got on with the job. I couldn't have had any nerves. In the final countdown, the championship officials still didn't want me in. I won nine out of ten races that season, and I probably only failed to clinch victory and a clean sweep in the last round at Donington Park because another guy torpedoed me into a crash.

Mick transferred all the preparation that he put into his own racing across to me. When I went to watch him, he used to climb in the back of his van and shout and yell and punch the hell out of the sides and doors. It's like he was completely psycho. Bloody scary to watch close-up, but it was his way of boosting himself for the challenge. He wanted my approach to racing to be as committed and I was a sponge, listening to him and absorbing all his psycho-babble intended to get me wound up and coiled for action. He made sure I was in the correct frame of mind – but I certainly didn't go to his extremes of thumping the van and screaming abuse at it. His value and his experience were immeasurable. He strove to instil race craft into me but, at the same time, insisted I did what came naturally to me and learn from my mistakes without repeating them. If I didn't learn, I'd risk a rollicking from him. He watched me like a hawk and worked hard at making me recognise the costly errors of silly mistakes, which were, in the main, down to my lack of experience.

I was an eager listener and learner and it paid off with good results. It made Mum pleased, too, that, like Ken before him, I had in Mick another influential figure to patiently steer me safely – even though she didn't really want me to go in that direction. Mick, despite his roguery, was a force for good so far as Mum was concerned, and it alleviated any scepticism she had initially harboured about his motives. He knew the business inside out and he got me to start thinking professionally about my racing attitude and preparation, even though I was still a schoolboy with all the uncertainties that go with it. He organised some sponsorship, which brought in a few pounds towards a van for the bikes, a mechanic and Bob and Dane to drive me to the circuits. All I had to do was ride the bike. I felt like a real racer. It all began to fit into place and the wins and records started to flow.

I reckoned I looked the part, very eye-catching, on an all-yellow bike with yellow leathers and my Arai helmet with a Union Jack painted over the top half. When you make that much of a spectacle of yourself, particularly in bright yellow, you have to be able to do the business or risk the jibes – all show, no go. It's a bit like footballers with their white boots or golfers with orange tartan trews and blue shoes. They have to deliver. I must have been a bit of an oddball, not only agreeing to ride glowing like a Caribbean sunburst or the world's biggest canary, but enjoying even the more mundane aspects of long journeys from home to racetracks down south. I had a lot to learn about the ways of racing. I enjoyed games such as the I-Spy games parents play with their bored kids on tedious car rides. Just past Junction 28 on the M1, on the left, is a field with a little tree standing on its own. One day with me, Mick, Bob and Dane in the van I blurted out, 'Oh, what a lovely little tree.' And all the others echoed mockingly, 'Oh, what a lovely little tree.' Afterwards, whenever we passed the spot, they would all take the piss, chorusing, 'Oh, what a lovely little tree.' I was supposed to be a hard-case biker, and all I could do was rattle on about the tree. Even now I wave to it. Is that sad or what?

Long journeys, jammed in vans with guys from your team, often right through the night, have a knack of throwing up odd and hilarious situations. As I became slowly absorbed into the world of racing, it was not only the racing legends that caught my attention; there were hundreds of stories and old anecdotes that accompanied them. They all played a part in luring me into the whole lifestyle. For example, one 'on the road' story I particularly remember is about Kenny Roberts, that great American rider. Years ago, before he had lots of money, he was travelling from his home in Modesto, California, in a van with his mechanic and a great friend, Bruce Cox, a lordly type of Englishman who lived in the USA. They were sitting three in a row across the front, with the mechanic driving and Bruce in the middle.

It was a long, tedious and tiring journey right across America and the mechanic, no doubt to keep himself awake, had one crack he kept repeating in his high-pitched and thoroughly grating voice. Whenever they were overtaken by a Greyhound bus, and this happened all the time through the night, the mechanic would yell,

'There goes the fastest animal in the WHOLE world.'
Kenny had just managed to slip off to sleep at 3 a.m. when
it happened again for what must have been about the
thousandth annoying time. Roberts, a bit short-tempered
at the best of times, was so irritated that he leaned across
Cox and smacked his mechanic in the mouth. That caused
the mechanic to lose control and swerve off the freeway
onto the verge, where the van stopped just a few feet away
from a highway patrol officer's chase car parked in the
middle of nowhere in the dead of night.

The officer was menacingly wearing sunglasses and was
about seven-feet tall, six-feet wide and mean-looking
under a hat with a brim so starched and stiff it looked like
a circular saw – and he was not best pleased.

Cox, the archetypal Englishman, superbly spoken with
a resonant voice and ever the diplomat, gestured to
Roberts, who was trying to shake the pain off his fist, and
the mechanic, now nursing his aching jaw, to sit tight
while he sorted matters out and placated the cop, who
was about to have reason to become even more curious.
The humidity in the Deep South was suffocating, even in
the early hours, and the sweating patrolman watched in
amazement as the portly, bushy-bearded figure of Cox
alighted from the van into the beam of his torch. He was
wearing a greenish three-piece heavy-tweed suit and a
bow tie – gear fit for an afternoon's tiffin after a shoot on
the Glorious Twelfth, but Alabama? Maybe not.

'My dear Constable, that's what we *very* respectfully
call you chaps where I come from,' greeted an unctuous
Cox, striving to impress the bewildered redneck with his
far-back and over-enunciated English accent, 'I'm sure we
can quickly resolve this unfortunate occurrence and we
will be about our business in a jiffy.'

Cox might have dropped in from a far planet, or at least
another part of America he had never heard of, so far as
the cop was concerned. He did not have a clue about the
accent until Cox explained he was from Britain and he
was in the company of one of the greatest of all American

motorbike aces on his way to race Daytona. The officer was impressed.

'So, we will be on our way, then?' inquired Cox.

'No, sir, indeedy no,' responded the policeman, 'aaaam gonna take you downtown.'

'Why on earth would you want to do that?' queried Cox.

'Because,' smiled the officer, 'I might have made history and arrested myself a fuckin' king here and the guys back at base would never believe it if I let you go.'

That tale of crazy America was a lesson for me to say that if mishaps could happen, they would, and you needed the strength of character to get through them. When I started out on the road, the stories could be a comfort at times. Not only was I learning how to develop a good yarn, I was also learning to deal with all the maturity and interdependence needed in the sport. I was getting absorbed into a supportive racing environment, but I could still feel desperately lonely at times. Once, when I was racing at Knockhill, that remotest of tracks, set in a very pituresque part of Scotland, I realised my life had turned into a roller coaster of emotions. I had been deeply affected by the deaths of my role models – my grandpa and my stepdad – and I had lost my base, my connection with two men who had been so crucial to my development.

I was doing OK in the races. I had qualified in sixth place, and should have been content with my lot as I guess most kids of my age would have been, but I was really quiet and generally withdrawn, did not mingle too much with the other riders and did not have many friends at the track. Mum was at home two hundred miles away and I felt extremely lost.

I always remember one night on track when I was walking on my own in the dark down to the start–finish line, looking at the countryside. It was a beautiful crystal-clear night, the stars were gleaming, the hills were far-off silhouettes reaching into the sky, and it seemed like another world of absolute peace far removed from the roar of rampaging racing motorbikes. I sat on the pit wall in the dark, feeling very sorry for myself. There were no sounds except the hum from the generators outside the teams' and riders' caravans. I looked up to the sky and cried. With tears streaming down my cheeks I wondered aloud if I would ever make it, would it ever happen for me, and how would I cope with the losses of the men I owed so much to. I had such a passion for my racing and I knew I could not possibly go it alone. And at sixteen you don't really know just what you are looking for amid all the confusion of growing up, but you realise you need something. I felt that everybody who had been such a motivating influence on my life had gone and wondered: who was up there? Who could I now turn to?

I sat there worrying about everything. Mum had been really struggling to fund my motorcycling until Mick Corrigan had come on the scene. It seemed I was living on a knife-edge, maybe not doing too well and not fulfilling any of the potential I promised, despite my eagerness. I was freezing, sitting on the edge of the track which the next day would be another and far different type of test. I didn't want to escape my little private communion with God or whoever just because I was shivering. I would have argued then that I was shivering with the cold, not the emotion, but now I think it was the latter.

Everything was happening so quickly. I had won the CB500 Newcomers' Cup and moved on to the CB500 National Cup. In the National 600 Championship I won by five seconds in the first race at Snetterton and moved up to the Supersports 600 Championship. In my first ever SS600 race at Brands Hatch I qualified eighth and finished fourth. Then, on the next round of SS600 at Thruxton, I qualified third and although I lost the front end while in the lead, it was because of a screw that got embedded in the flat front Dunlop of my bike. Although most people would see that rate of progress as an achievement, I was worried that critics would be thinking I was nothing new

– fast guys come and fast guys go, don't they? I was sixteen years and nine months old – a school kid. However, Italians such as Loris Capirossi, who was the youngest ever world champion at seventeen, have been successful at an early age, and Ivan Goi and Valentino Rossi have even won Grand Prix events aged sixteen.

I was also already having to cope with the press coverage that accompanies the sport. My mum has assiduously, and typically neatly, kept press and magazine cuttings tracking my career right from the beginning, and they seemed to have reached avalanche levels from the moment Mick Corrigan took, and tucked, me under his wing.

It is amazing to me now when I browse through the albums how much faith was put in my ability and, at the time, how unaware I was about the hype I seemed to have attracted. It is as if all the fuss about my achievements were about somebody else, another kid who appeared to be doing wondrous things on a motorbike. All I was doing, if my memory serves me right, was enjoying myself without thinking too hard or deeply about the effect I was having on the rest of racing.

There is one magazine article that even now makes me blush with embarrassment at its unashamedly laudatory tone. I suppose, and this is what Mum says, they were only writing what they believed to be a true opinion and an honest appraisal of the way they thought my career was heading. And in that respect, I should be grateful that some people took time to write nice things about me. In *Superbike* under the heading 'The Super Teen' and with the strapline 'Could This Lad Be The Fastest Teenager Britain's Ever Seen?' there was a main picture of me leading those great Isle of Man TT winners and heroes, Jim Moodie and Phillip McCallen and the champion Dave Heal, in a downpour at Brands Hatch in my first ever British Supersport race in 1997. It reads: 'James Toseland. Remember this name if you've never heard of him before. If you're a regular at National and UK Superbike race meetings the name will be familiar enough.'

My name would have been familiar merely because they tend to namecheck the leaders fairly often irrespective of what class is on track at the time. I had been in a few classes and at the front of most of them that year. I think, of course, there was added interest in me from the beginning because I was British. I was described, flatteringly, as being very mature for my age, but Mick had to fight to bypass the regulations all the way. Rules could have easily prevented me from racing with these older boys until I'd got my exam results back, not while I was in the middle of sitting them. I guess I seemed a lot more mature than the average teenager to those in the business. However, my youth did come across very strongly at other times. I did a Question and Answer session with *Superbike*, too; they called it 'The Voice of Youth'.

Q: What is more important, school or racing?
A: Exams count, but racing comes first every time.
Q: Who's your ideal woman?
A: To be honest, I'm not fussed.

I think nowadays I might have a different response, a bit more damningly revealing, to questions about women. Issues have assumed a different level of importance as I have grown to appreciate the benefits, shall we say, that come from being upfront as a motorbike racer and a world champion.

I don't see any reason why, if they've got their heads about them, the next generation of young bikers shouldn't come through the system without the licence wrangles I had to overcome. I was asked about it at the time and recommended that the ruling bodies take a good look at what younger riders are achieving in this country. Us Brits don't dare to chuck our young riders in at the deep end. Valentino Rossi was thrown into GPs and look what he's done. He is only doing what he does now because he got to ride with the best in the world at an early age – that and a lot of talent, of course. I was chucked into the deep end and I can only get quicker now. If young talent is staying in classes where they are winning, the riders don't have to get any quicker because they are winning already. There is a lot of good talent out there, but it should be pushed to go for the big time.

My GCSEs were a bit disrupted by the racing, and I could and should have done better, but there was so much happening in my life with the bike racing coming together that I was being deflected from schoolwork. It's easy to say this now, but I don't expect I was thinking quite so deeply when, in 1997, I was sitting my GCSEs and racing at Brands Hatch. I had a cookery test at school in Yorkshire on a Friday morning; and a qualifying session at the Kent track, 200-odd miles south, in the afternoon. Neither time could be changed, so I had to do both in one day. Mick's brother Bob rode up on a motorbike and waited at the school gates for me. I did the exam and sprinted out, still in my school uniform, for a quick zoom to Brands on the pillion.

Mick was never shy in singing my praises and would say to every challenger, 'James is going to be world champion one day. He's a star. He will go all the way.'

His prophecy was as much a challenge to me as it was an acclamation.

Racing as I was, at the highest level in the UK, I was up against a set of lads who had gained fame at places as different as the Isle of Man and all the really testing short circuits such as Brands Hatch, Cadwell Park, Mallory, Oulton and Knockhill in Scotland – places that were mostly new to me when I had moved up the classes to take on the big boys in the British championships. However, I honestly never felt as if I was struggling: quite the opposite at times. Without wanting to sound big-headed, I was being held up by them. I did not think I was being, or doing, anything extra-special. I was just riding the bike as best I could. And here I was, not just holding my own, but getting the better of some really good and quick guys who had loads of experience, on a really good bike.

I was also being well looked after by Mick Corrigan and the team and my confidence was at a peak. So much so that I reckoned the competition was not a problem. I did not sense any jealousy, nothing that has followed me as a bad memory down the years. I guess it was because I had arrived on the scene as a raw youngster, well wet behind the ears, and nobody could, or wanted to, criticise me because I was only a kid trying to do his best. Being beaten by a spotty little kid like me could not have been the most enjoyable experience for some of the guys who had been around a while, but if they did take it badly nobody let me know. I knew how to ride a bike – and ride it safely – and I was doing well, which seemed to please rather than anger or irritate people. I wasn't treading on anybody's toes, riding like a madman or pulling all the women – that would really have upset some of them. I was just a sixteen-year-old lad out for a good time.

It is really bizarre to look back at all those old pages and headlines from the likes of *Motorcycle News* and see myself described variously as a 'sensation', 'teenage won-derboy', 'super-starlet', and 'sure-fire world champion of the future'. I had won five of the last six races in the British 600 championship, having started the series when it was already halfway through and I was still at school. It is a wonder that I managed to stay on an even keel without going overboard or becoming unbearably con-ceited. I put all that ability to stay clear-headed and unaffected down to all the teachings I had been given and an eagerness to listen and learn.

There have been many more comments made about me, good, bad and indifferent, and I have tried to deal with each one on its merits without either being chuffed or angry according to its tone. I argue you cannot please all of the people all of the time. Not very original, but true. The deepest newspaper articles seem to hit the spot, not just because they might be praiseworthy, but more because they manage to transmit some of my own thoughts, too. Everybody needs levels of encouragement and if I had not had people backing me, and subsequent support from Mum, Grandpa Alec and all the family, Ken and Mick, then my name as a racing motorcyclist would not have existed. We just didn't have the resources to sustain my ambitions and I would have had to stop. Luck, too, plays such a crucial role and, when it comes your way, you have to make sure you are ready to take advantage. Mix the two together, the interest that others have in you, and that little bit of good fortune, and you should be onto a winner. What else could get in my way?

One of the proudest moments I remember – and it still gives me a little buzz – was that partway through the 1997 season, I had a one-off race on a Fireblade, that real beast of a bike, just for fun. I managed just one test session at Mallory Park, finished an amazing fourth in the race and beat Ian Simpson, a superb rider, who won the title that year. Then, I followed it up with an embarrassing episode to prove that there is always an underlying threat to bring you back down to earth with a bang. I fell off in a big way doing a wacky, show-off wheelie in front of a big crowd at Brands Hatch at the end of what had been a fantastic season. Race officials fined me £800 for the celebration that went wrong – and thought seriously about docking my points for the win.

Towards the end of my time with Mick Corrigan's team, when I started winning, I suddenly found myself in the money. Mick let me keep the prize money. £800 a time for winning a race and £800 for winning the 600 Championship. Not bad for a sixteen-year-old – and, don't forget, I had won the last five out of six races. I felt like I had scooped the lottery. I made up my mind to give Mum a treat by way of thanks for all her help and sacrifice as soon as I had accumulated enough to spring a decent and memorable surprise.

I clinched the national CB500 1997 title with Mick's team at Knockhill in Scotland with three races of the championship still to go. I also had a second victory in the Supersport 600 series to add to my successes. Two days later, there was some news. Honda (yes, HONDA of all teams) wanted to put me on a Castrol-backed CBR600 with a deal to race in the World Supersport championship. Talk about being happy and excited. I was sixteen and I'd had more than eleven firm offers, including a £250,000 deal for a 125 Grand Prix ride, for the 1998 season and now I had a three-year deal with Honda.

I jacked in the paper delivery round.

Neil Tuxworth, an ex-TT rider, very persuasive and a real toughie, was the Castrol–Honda team manager. He was pleased to offer me the natural progression because he believed I needed and deserved it for what had been an impressive debut season.

After the super year I'd had with Mick Corrigan in 1997, some ten wins on the 500 and a sensational spell beating Britain's best on the 600 halfway through the season at sixteen years of age, I moved into the whirlwind experience of racing in the World Supersport series with Castrol–Honda. I went from battling it out with the finest home-based guys to taking on experienced international riders on a much wider stage, with even greater expectation and pressure put on me. I didn't mind. I didn't understand the magnitude of it all and at that age (I was then seventeen) my view was that I was just mixing with a different set of people who spoke languages I didn't or couldn't follow. On the bike, it didn't matter what language anybody spoke.

My improvement had been so dramatic and so quick, and with the fabulous and irresistible offer from Castrol–Honda in the pipeline, the time was ripe for me, reluctantly but with everlasting gratitude, to move out of Mick's control and become a works rider, every pro biker's dream. It had begun to dawn on me, not because of what people were so kindly saying or writing about me, but more because of what I was achieving, that I was more than just another rider. Underneath it all, I was still puzzled and found it difficult to understand what all the fuss was about. To me, I was simply doing what came naturally. Racing. And winning.

Four

RIDE THE WILD WIND

There is not a rider out there who, in the event of his death while doing his damnedest for the team, would not want everyone else to continue. We all accept that getting hurt, crippled sometimes and, thank God less frequently, killed, goes hand in hand with being a motorbike racer.

For the first round of the 1998 series at Donington Park it snowed. And I fell off, over the high-side, on lap two. Welcome to World Supersport racing . . .

It was a case of getting straight back on again for round two at Monza, that super-fast and historic track with its five left-hand and eight right-hand corners, and never-ending straight. In Friday qualifying, I came off the bike, in a very painful way – and it was all because I did not have the experience of warming the tyres up to a favourable temperature. I was feeling under a lot of pressure and was desperate to do well after my crash at Donington Park. I remember thinking: I have to pull myself together and put all this behind me. I was hardly pushing the bike at all because I wanted to get to know the circuit better before I got up to speed and really went for it. Then, the unthinkable happened. I belted out of the chicane onto the back straight into a quick left-hander – and the bike suddenly squirmed, dug in and threw me over the handlebars. It somersaulted and landed on me, then kept rolling and dragged me, still pinned by its weight (about 165 kg), down the track. Both my ankles snapped under the impact. I was in agony and realised this was a nasty one. I couldn't free myself and a marshal had to heave the bike off me.

Up until then I had never broken a bone, not even the tiniest crack, so I didn't have any realisation of just how painful it was going to get before I could be transferred to the medical centre for treatment. Two shattered ankles were a real introduction to the business of broken bones and how to cope with such a huge setback. To make my frustration and anxiety worse, I was not allowed to fly back to Britain because the swelling in my legs could have turned thrombotic and the surgeon ruled it was too dangerous.

I had to be driven back that evening in the team's motorhome with both my legs in plaster. It was a strange and lonely trip. It took two thoroughly miserable days with me stretched out on a sofa and feeling very gloomy and sorry for myself. To say nothing of the pain – and, of course, the worry at the back of my mind that I might be so badly screwed up that I would never race again.

The experience really tested my bravado and made me realise how easily riders can get complacent. To be the ultimate, unbeatable racer and the champion of champions is not just a goal, it is a belief. Without such ambition, without the eagerness to play catch-up with distant aims, we are nothing.

My hero, that truly amazing Tour de France legend Lance Armstrong, is a perfect example. In fact, look at any sportsman, any world champion, and most have at sometime in their life had to master downsides that have put their drive to be a winner to the test, only for them to triumph spectacularly and deservedly. When you want something so much, it is not very difficult to motivate yourself. At least, that's what I have found: getting myself into the right frame of mind for any challenge has always been second nature to me. The things that happened to my family left me with a resolve and a positive outlook. What loved ones passed on to me was a gift to be able to turn every setback into a positive and to draw strength from adversity. That has carried over into my racing. I am ferociously competitive, aggressive and always ready to overturn situations that would otherwise, and with most people, wreck hope and destroy dreams.

When we finally got home, we pulled up outside Mum's house. She was crying when she saw the state I was in with the mechanic carrying me in like a helpless child. And just as I was trying to deal with that, my brother blurted out, 'Your team-mate has been killed.' I could not believe what I was hearing and asked him to make sure he had got the right rider and to check out the guy's name: Michael Paquay.

Simon was correct. Michael was dead. This lovely fellow, a real golden rider and an awesome guy of only 24, my team-mate for just two rounds, had died in another really high-speed crash the day after mine. He was hurtling down the long start-and-finish straight trying to make up for the Honda's lack of competitive speed by slipstreaming a rider in front. But he got too close and clipped the other guy's back wheel. Inevitably at such a fast rate of knots, he crashed.

As the news came through, I was heartbroken by the details. Michael clipped the rear of another bike on the fastest part of the Monza course, where speeds reach up to 165 mph. He was flung into the path of French rider Sebastien Charpentier and Italian Ferdinando Di Maso and both their bikes hit Paquay, causing massive internal injuries. I cannot imagine the trauma his loved ones must have felt as the race doctors battled to restart his heart and stabilise him. Michael was rushed to a nearby Monza hospital that was equipped to deal with Formula One racing-car accidents, but even though medics battled to save him, giving him artificial respiration for 45 minutes after his heart gave out, he died while he was being operated on. It was a dreadful tragedy and a great shame because he was a brilliant prospect and looked a sure-fire world champion.

I wince now when I thumb through Mum's album and see the *Motorcycle News* pictures of me being carried by two guys out of the trackside medical centre with both legs encased in plaster up to my knees. But it is a far more painful memory to see photos of Paquay, looking so neat and tidy and fit in his white leathers, across the page and a wonderful last shot of him in spectacular action with his knee scraping the ground on a really high-speed corner.

It makes me feel incredibly selfish to think of it, but at the time I was feeling quite sorry for myself with my injuries. I was at home facing a race against time to be fit for the German round in four weeks' time. I had been told by doctors not to walk for two weeks. I was gutted and sank into a good long period of utter despondence. With all the irrational doubts of a seventeen-year-old, my main worry was that my career could be ebbing away before it had got into full flow. I just wanted to get back on the bike as soon as I could, to show that all the faith people had put in my ability was not misplaced and I was not a careless crasher.

I couldn't believe that I had been there while it was all happening. It hit me that I was one very lucky guy. Michael, who I had met only a couple of times and did not know too well, had been killed and I had got away with a pretty big bang. A lot of people over the years, really superb riders, have died crashing, but you never think it is going to happen to you. I suppose that toweringly high level of confidence that you are fireproof, false though it may be, was underpinned by my own lucky escape. If smashing both ankles can be regarded as a lucky escape . . .

In two days the Castrol–Honda team had suffered two major blows. My problems, as bad as I felt, were nothing compared with the awful accident that had befallen my friend. Everyone was so deeply moved by the crash, which was officially classified as a racing accident. Flags at the track were flown half-mast and scores of riders and team staff wore black armbands as a mark of respect. Paquay's untimely death was a tremendous blow to the team and under those circumstances it is almost impossible to justify what, to outsiders, must seem like heartless decisions to carry on. However, there is not a rider who, in the event of his death while he was doing his damnedest for the team, would not want everyone else to continue. We all accept that getting hurt, crippled sometimes and, thank God less frequently, killed, goes hand in hand with being a motorbike racer. And, therefore, Neil Tuxworth, the team boss, announced that Castrol–Honda would continue:

'We will go on. Michael would not want us to pull out. First and foremost he was a racer and the best way for us to honour him is to try and achieve something positive,' he said.

As the team were pushing on I knew once again that I would have to force myself to push through the pain. It was a strange feeling going straight from another tragedy, back to the track – I was used now to the strange detached feeling of letting myself be caught up in another world, switching off and concentrating all my energy on the races. It would be sometime before any decision was made about a possible replacement for Paquay. We missed the next round of the championship in Albacete in Spain the next week because, of course, I was also out, but they did say they would continue with me when I was fit.

Six weeks later I abandoned the wheelchair and, trying to hide the pain, hobbled on my hardly mended ankles for a comeback at Misano, on Italy's Adriatic coast. It was not the greatest idea I'd ever had, but an unwise impatience and desperation to get back into action drove me to want to push myself beyond the limits. It was a risk too far. Or was it stupidity? Anyway, two days after I got out of my wheelchair, I rode in qualifying for the Supersport race. I could not get closer than three and a half seconds to the pole-man, an Italian, Vito Guareschi, who was all fired up to win on home ground. That left me down among the also-rans in a very lowly, very embarrassing fortieth place, with only 36 riders allowed on the grid.

I just could not get up to competitive speed, the pain from my ankles was too much to bear and it affected my concentration, my physical capacity to work the controls and just about everything else. I knew it wasn't going to be easy, but my fitness was so far gone that I didn't have the strength to do better. I had been sitting on my arse in a wheelchair for six weeks and my ankles were in agony. I couldn't put pressure on the pegs to make the bike turn fast enough. Even so, Neil Tuxworth, I guess because he had been a top-class rider himself and appreciated the problems we all face getting back from injury, was as supportive as ever and he said I had done very well just to be there. He said that if I had tried to go too fast I would have risked aggravating the injury.

I picked up the pace again with a tenth place in the next round in South Africa – and, after all the crashes and misfortunes that had blighted my start in the Supersport championship, I was well relieved to bring the bike home in Kyalami with us both in one piece. Eighths, ninths and tenths followed and I was riding well within myself, determined to keep Honda happy. Nothing spectacular, no balls-out and chancy attempts to win, just carefully controlled effort. It paid off because Neil announced they were hanging on to me for 1999 despite what he described as 'James's nightmare debut season in international racing'.

I found I had two minders in my colleagues from the Castrol–Honda Superbike team Aaron Slight and Colin Edwards who were always quick to fly to my defence. At a press conference, when the questions about my first season were getting a little too probing and unsympathetic for their liking, Colin, angry on my behalf, grabbed the microphone and snarled, 'Get off his back. Let him get on with his job.' It was yet another graphic indication of their support for me. And, honestly, the pair of them were an inspiration and an encouragement when I needed it the most.

The piano playing began to tail off when Honda approached me. With all the travelling and the time I had to put into testing and racing and promotional activities I couldn't keep up with the routine lessons. I had reached a stage where I was playing really well. I was now able to sight-read and I was enjoying my music. However, I knew there was nothing I wanted more in life than to be a racer. I got up to Grade 6 at the piano and if I had continued onto Grade 8 I would have been able to interview at the college in London. That would have pleased Mum no end. But I am afraid the only grade I was really interested in was being Number One on two wheels.

Any ideas that I may have harboured, in deference to my mum's preferences, to go to the London College of Music and become a pro piano player in an orchestra were blown right out of my thoughts. I can imagine how her fears for my safety were accelerated. But she had known all along that I wasn't going to be shaken away from my stubborn goal. She realised how much I wanted it. That's why, whatever her innermost doubts, she supported me. If she had not backed me all the way with such selfless personal and financial sacrifice as she did, I don't think she could have lived with herself. That's the way she is.

Obviously, I did not completely abandon the piano. It continued to be a way of breaking free from the tensions and into a haven of relaxation. I still play to wind down after races because, in many ways, the instrument has been a vent to my pent-up emotions and jamming away on it can induce an almost soporific level of escapism. It works the other way, too. When I feel exhilarated I want to lift the lid and give freedom to my personal satisfaction with happier tunes to fit my upbeat mood. A lot of sportsmen have no other outlets when the tensions, pre- and post-event, make demands on their concentration, so they can plunge into all sorts of trouble. People often ask me if I worry that I may crash heavily enough to damage my hands so badly that I could never play the piano again, but honestly, I never think about it. I guess it would upset me if I was hurt badly enough and, say, lost a couple of fingers or something, which meant I couldn't play. I have hit the tarmac a couple of times and taken off the end of a thumb and then smashed a bone in my hand, but never with enough damage to restrict my playing.

I know some people cannot understand the parallels of being a so-called hard-case, daredevil racing motorcyclist and a pianist with a serious, artistic interest in music. They don't seem to be able to twig the connection. This lack of appreciation that the two passions can live happily together, as if playing the piano were some wimpish betrayal of biking, was laughably demonstrated at Brands Hatch, on a phenomenal day in 2003. It was when I was racing against everybody's hero, my pal Neil Hodgson, a homely lad from Burnley, Lancashire, and soon to be crowned World Superbike champion, with me third in the final countdown which took place in front of a jam-packed 120,000 crowd. Before the race, I spotted this massive banner: 'Hodgson's No Pianist – He's World Champion', as if playing the piano rendered me a no-hoper and disqualified me as a title contender. Whoever that creative person was – and there was really a lot of work put in behind the banner having a dig at me – they evidently believed that a pianist can't be a motorcyclist or a champion, because biking has the macho image that piano playing does not. Anyway, I decided to show them. In the opener Neil was second to my sixth place with wild card Shane Byrne, the British champ, grabbing a double in the two-leg European round. But in the second outing, I had my revenge: I was third with Hodgy behind me in fifth place.

After the tough 1998 season, and all the pain that went with it, I was even more determined to make it to the top in motorbike racing. In fact, the pain made me desperate to succeed and use my disappointment to spur what I can only describe as a basic drive to be the best. I knew deep down inside that if I could hold on to my ambitions after such an eventful and threatening start to my international career, I should be OK. I decided to concentrate on Neil Tuxworth's and Honda's trust in my ability, which never wavered even though I reckoned my talent had only barely begun to show. There were enough knowing, well-meaning and experienced people behind me to keep me following an upward curve and I wanted to do them justice. I am not ashamed to keep emphasising it, but my mum was again the biggest help at this stage. While a lot of my new-found maturity was down to my own strength of character, there were times when I was alone in a hotel room thousands of miles from anywhere and everything was going wrong, and all I wanted to do was talk to my mum. She would always take the time to listen to me when I rang and she was absolutely faultless in her support. Colin Edwards and Aaron Slight were fantastic support, and my manager Neil Tuxworth was brilliant, but there's nobody like Mum.

I forced myself through a gruelling get-fitter regime that would have seriously tested an Olympic athlete. After I had smashed my ankles in the Monza crash, being confined to a wheelchair for four weeks naturally sent my fitness levels into a nosedive. Just as soon as I could get out of the plaster casts and back onto my feet I hit the gymnasium for three to four hours a day, every day. I was rowing, running, riding and weightlifting with such commitment it was scary. I blocked out all the tiredness and boredom of sitting on an exercise bike by imagining that I was in a race, dicing with the front-runners. Sometimes I drove myself to extreme exhaustion levels, but I wouldn't let myself give in. Whatever the discomfort, I just kept trying to focus on the benefits that super-fitness would give me.

I remember seeing an article about the great champion Mick Doohan's superman state of fitness, how on comprehensively analysed tests he could outperform footballers, tennis players, boxers and all sorts of athletes, and all with a heartbeat so slowed down it was hardly ticking over. He was rated one of the fittest sportsmen on the planet and that was my target, too. He was the picture, the ideal role model whenever I began to flag or falter. And it all worked. I underwent months of training in preparation for the 1999 season and I was raring to go. I was lucky that I realised just how crucial it is to be both mentally and physically attuned and fit to be a winner. I look at great riders such as Mick Doohan and I know that is how dedicated you need to be to become the best in the world. I have a job to do that I love – and to keep fit enough to do it is no big deal for me. Sometimes I can hardly believe that I am being paid to do the thing I love most in the world – race motorbikes.

A lot of people felt that after the events of 1998, some riders would have retired or taken a year out, but I had made myself stronger and kept things in perspective. And that made me think positively – I was back with a far more mature head on my shoulders. Talk about meaning business. I remember that recognition of my own will to win, no matter what was written about me, and it has never left me since. I get a kick now when I look back at the season and yet still find it difficult to appreciate that it was me that everyone said all those admiring words about. People forgot that I was just seventeen in my first international season and seventeen-year-olds do things that maybe they shouldn't do in a race. I was determined that this year was going to be different – I was no longer a kid.

Just before the 1999 season opened, under the headline 'I'm Not a Child Any More' and, beside a photograph that made me look like a school prefect who hadn't yet started shaving, I gave my considered opinions about the upcoming Supersport campaign under the Castrol–Honda banner. The feature cited the torrid time I'd had crashing out of my first World Supersport 600 race at Donington Park after my 'meteoric rise to stardom' then the Monza disaster with Michael Paquay's death and my injuries. It also referred to me 'not living up to expectations' and those last remarks hurt.

I kept my confidence levels high throughout the pre-season, but it was another matter being back out on the circuit and surrounded by the cream of the crop. I remember Neil Tuxworth, a well-respected Grand Prix and Isle of Man TT rider, took me to one side and insisted, 'Look, plenty of great guys have been through really bad times before they got to the top ... brilliant riders like Kevin Schwantz, Mick Doohan and Luca Cadalora ... they have all had terrible years like yours ... and they have all survived as much stronger men. So can you.'

Neil's reminder cleared away any lingering doubts and made me appreciate what I had achieved: I had gone from being in the CB500 Cup at home to the World Supersport 600 series in just eight months. It was a massive leap onto a vast international stage to face competition from some fast and competent riders destined for greater things and hell-bent on doing their darnedest to get there. I had learned so much that I could take into this next new season and it would make me a better rider. For example, I am honoured to have become a member of a small, but elite, band of motorbike race champions and flattered to the point of embarrassment whenever I am recognised. If that is the price of success, then I am quite happy to put up with it and I would hope that if it ever appears to be going to my head then somebody would do me the great favour of telling me. The bottom line, and this really is the crux of racing success, is that once you are on the bike in a madcap crush of other guys, all going at 200 mph, all as ferociously motivated as you are to win and refusing to yield an inch – there is nobody to help you. You are on your own. Confidence and ability – and, of course, a good, fast, reliable bike – are the essentials you need to work right on the edge of survival and safety. Having said that, they are nothing without an in-built determination to overcome the odds by being daring but not reckless, wary but not fearful, and so single-minded you can visualise only victory until the dictates of the race shape it otherwise.

Although I enjoy listening and learning from people, I find it hard to rely on others. When you have nobody to blame but yourself for any shortcomings then you guarantee, as far as humanly possible, not to make any blunders or take stupid chances. I suppose it is that state of mind, a totally singular outlook that gives me the focus I crave to be a success at whatever I do.

It sounds selfish I know, but I realised early on that I had to be focused and diversions, when there might be somebody else's feelings and concerns to be considered, was not the right way for me. I have had only three serious girlfriends and each one lasted about two years – between times it has just been a case of having fun with good-time not long-time girls. I think I always expected that the way my career was going, serious considerations such as girlfriends would stand in the way of success. Having said that, I did get engaged when I was eighteen, a foolish and rather rash move that seemed a good idea at the time, to only the second girlfriend I'd ever had. It happened six months after we met. She was a student, a stunning-looking lass – and still is – from Sheffield. The engagement, though I don't think we ever discussed getting married, came about simply because my brother had got engaged and I thought if our kid has done it then it must be the fashionable thing to do. He is still with his lady, Kirsty, and they have two brilliant children. Jenny and me lasted about eighteen months. My ex-fiancée is now a successful radiologist.

I don't want to get too deep about this, but the Toseland Rules of Relationships seems to hark back to my days as a kid growing up with a mum who regarded herself as a single mother. She always warned me not to get hooked up with relationships. It was something she drilled into me: don't get involved, you cannot cut off your emotions, so don't let them get in a tangle.

To date I haven't met the right girl, or come even close to believing I have. I thought I had at 18 – but the changes and attitudes that overtake you by the time you get to the age I am now at the time of writing, 24, are totally unpredictable. If I had gone through with my engagement

I guess it would have been completely the wrong thing to do and two peoples' lives, Jenny's and mine, could have been ruined.

Five

I WANT IT ALL

It is a conscious decision to push yourself as far as you dare, while still keeping your fate firmly in your own hands. I think every full-blooded racer, on bikes or in cars, shares that wonderful exciting sensation.

With the stream of good advice and genuine support I was receiving, I went into the Kyalami race in South Africa for the 1999 World Supersport championship with a sensible attitude. I resisted the temptation of a win-or-crash dash. I had qualified seventeenth, which put me on the fifth row of the grid, and the bike had some suspension problems and was running lean because of the high altitude and the thinner air, so I wasn't exactly in the ideal situation. I was chasing the local hero, Russell Wood, and I guess I could have given him a harder time, but, equally, I could have embarrassingly legged-off again and that would not have pleased anybody – mostly myself. So I sat tight, played a safe game and harvested ten points for a career-best result of sixth place. Instead of getting all worked up and stupidly going for a higher finish, I coasted home in one piece for the points. I was dubbed 'Mr Sensible' after that. My new Supersport team-mate, the Spaniard Pere Riba crashed on the last lap of the 23 and I was left to fly the Castrol–Honda flag.

There were no wins that season, but it turned into something of a showcase for me with some really good and eye-catching rides leading to points-scoring places with fightbacks from low qualifying positions: an eighth from fifteenth on the grid in front of 50,000 at Donington Park, my home track; then a thirteenth from the very back and thirtieth fastest on a troublesome bike, in the teeming rain in Misano, Italy; there was an eleventh from twenty-sixth place in qualifying in Albacete, Spain; and another eleventh at Laguna Seca, California. These and some other good, hard-going scraps for places got me up to eleventh place in the championship.

I still get goosebumps now when I recall the reception I got at Brands Hatch that year. There were more than 100,000 people packed into the Kent circuit for what was a major event and the support, the buzz and the constant attention was unbelievable. I was certainly made to feel that I had arrived on the racing scene with colourful banners and flags bearing my name everywhere. With my name being touted alongside racing legend Carl Fogarty, I was motivated like never before to give the race my best shot. All of my team-mates were doing their best to boost my confidence and the principals of the team were so strong that I had this extra edge – an anxiety to succeed.

As I set off, there was this intense fascination and magic as I felt I was taking a bike right to the edge, and the fact that I was surviving out there on the track filled me with this heightened sense of satisfaction. I would never describe it as like being on a drug. Drug-taking could never be for me because it is all about losing control of your senses, whereas this feeling was an irresistible urge to overcome and master self-doubt. I had full control and even though I couldn't get any closer, as hard as I tried, to the front-runners I got a seventh place in the 23-lapper and I was happy enough.

Some sportsmen I know take drugs or drink themselves silly because they can't live without the pedestal of emotion they put themselves on, so when the attention they crave falters they resort to these very sickening alternatives. But I react far differently. I honestly do not want or need that intensity of celebrity and all the ballyhoo that goes with it. I prefer to relax in a normal state well away from the environment that can give you such a false impression of your own importance. If, after the end of the season when you have finished racing, when all the worldwide attention you were subject to ebbs away, you pine for it and miss it and you feel robbed because the afterglow has dimmed, then I don't believe that is a healthy state of mind to be in.

The ex-champion Formula One driver Jacques Villeneuve, as brave a driver as they come, always reckons that existing on the threshold, sometimes crossing it and surviving, is a feeling that cannot be transmitted and understood by others who have never experienced it. He revels in the sheer exhilaration of blasting flat out in top gear through the awesomely scary and tricky Eau Rouge section at Spa in the Belgian Ardennes. He says:

Spa is an amazing place to go racing. It is like a wild roller-coaster ride that takes your breath away. It is the driving experience of a lifetime.

The car jumps sideways with sparks flying, you're fighting the wheel, hanging on as best you can with vision blurred from all the bouncing, the engine screaming more loudly than ever in your ears and you have to keep your mind set on doing what seems impossible: taking Eau Rouge flat out.

You have to make a conscious decision to do it. You have to break through a barrier that is mental as well as physical.

When you are going flat out there it seems like you are climbing straight up into the sky. You're turning left and right while the car gets very heavy and flattens itself down on the track because of the extra downforce, but the adhesion is precarious and the car skips sideways . . . at about 300 kph. Even if you feel you are on the verge of disaster you have to imagine your right foot is bolted to the floor and you cannot lift off. You have to tell yourself 'My foot is not coming up' and you hang on in there, getting more and more tense. You stop breathing. You start to close your eyes. NO, you DON'T close your eyes. They stay wide open . . . with fear. But when you are safely through Eau Rouge you blink rapidly. The thrill is tremendous.

The first time you successfully take Eau Rouge flat out you wonder if you should ever tempt fate again. You feel as if you have been right on the ragged edge and maybe you were lucky to make it. A lot of what happens there depends on instinct and blind faith in your own capabilities. The problem with being so much on the limit through there is that you are in less control of a situation in which the car is fully stressed. And so are you.

Villeneuve has always insisted that there is nowhere he prefers more to be than on the edge – as close to going over it as he dares. It is not a death wish. It is a conscious decision to push yourself as far as you dare, while still keeping your fate firmly in your own hands. I think every full-blooded racer, on bikes or in cars, shares that wonderful exciting sensation. This sport can really get under your skin. It keeps you throbbing with intensity, a crucial element when you are confronted and surrounded by around 25 equally gifted, world-class riders, none of whom would willingly yield one millimetre of track, in the madcap melee that sums up racing on two wheels.

The 1998 and 1999 seasons were a difficult couple of years because the Honda was not really competitive, but I had further fears about my career. I worried that I was about to find out that I may have to return from World Supersport to the British championship – and that would be a difficult pill to swallow. I went to the motorcycle show at the NEC in Birmingham and met up with Roger Harvey, the Honda-UK race manager. Something must have clicked deep down inside me, I don't know what, but I suspected I might be on the brink of being jettisoned from the World Supersport line-up, so I asked him straight out, 'Have I got a job – or not? I'm not at all sure. Can you find out for me?'

He called Neil Tuxworth, the team manager, and the fact that he was not smiling when he came off the phone gave me my clue. He said I was out and he explained they wanted me to return to the British Supersport championship, doing again at nineteen what I had already done at sixteen. I was really pissed off and I said that if I was coming back to a British championship I wanted to move up to Superbike and not return to Supersport. I had been there, done that and could not see any advantage or advancement for my career. 'Give me a chance,' I said, 'I've finished the job in Supersport, now I want to go upwards.'

I felt I was still able to ride and race OK and I was still on the up. I ended up slotting into Paul Bird's British Superbike team, a fantastic set-up, even if we did have only one Honda and the rival Harris team had two. The way they looked after me at my age and level of experience was brilliant. Moving across to Castrol–Honda under Neil Tuxworth's guidance was a significant step forwards, for which I was grateful. I had, in return, given them everything I could. It upset me that they dragged their feet in offering me the chance of promotion up to World Superbike level. If they had I would have happily put pen to paper.

As it turned out, if I had persuaded Honda to give me another deal, as I thought they would have done halfway through the 1999 season when I was riding pretty well, I would have been tied to them and would not have been available to take up the fabulous offer that was being mooted without my being aware.

I went through to the 2000 season, having signed to ride the Demon Vimto Honda in the British Superbike championships, but I was experiencing only modest results, far below my own hopes and dreams, and I felt I was trapped in a cycle of crashes, tyre problems and consistently tough struggles against the very experienced likes of Steve Hislop, John Reynolds, Chris Walker, Neil Hodgson, James Haydon and old-stager Niall Mackenzie.

In my first ever race aboard the VTR1000 SP1 Honda Superbike at Brands Hatch in March 2000, I got off to a really slow start, a bit uncharacteristic for me then, and had to play catch-up from seventeenth place. Even though I was racing on slicks for the first time I managed to get by Michael Rutter and Paul Young's Level Three Yamahas and then Sean Emmett with two laps left for an eleventh place. I wasn't too unhappy with that but I sensed I would be able to do much better as I got more used to the bike. I'm sure I could have run a lot nearer the front had I got off to a better start, but it was good experience as I was learning all the time. My new boss, Paul Bird, said at the time that it was a good result for us under the circumstances. We had to make a lot of changes to the suspension, but we were making good strides and he seemed confident that I would soon be on the pace. After just seven races Paul confirmed that he wanted to keep me on for 2001, and he was pestering Honda-Britain to order full-blown works bikes with guaranteed backing money from Vimto and the Internet company Demon to pay for them. I and the other Honda riders were campaigning on SP-1s, which had been modified with a range of parts. Paul announced to the press: 'I've got the money sorted out for the full works kit, but the only rider I want is James Toseland.'

The season ebbed unhappily and disappointingly to an early conclusion with ups and down in equal measure: a crash at Snetterton, getting knocked off at Silverstone, a pretty good seventh in the first leg at Oulton Park, a better sixth in the second leg, and an enforced drop-out with tyre problems at Thruxton. I came an overall seventh place in the championship. It was all a test of my character as a budding professional and showed my eagerness to take the inevitable rough with the infrequent smooth.

Then, to my horror, I went upside down ... again ... in a spectacular crash testing at Cadwell Park. And, once again, I finished up with broken bones. This time my femur was shattered in three places. I missed the last five rounds, and a World Superbike wild-card entry at Brands Hatch – a real heartbreaker because I was so desperate to show myself as a potential champion – but I was still the highest-placed Honda man in the British series.

I remember sitting alone at home, leg in plaster, and wondering if I had wrecked my career, because you never know what complications can set in with fractures as bad as that was. That, of course, and being out of the limelight for another extended spell when you can be easily forgotten or overlooked, made me fear that any opportunity I had made for myself would be offered to somebody else.

My mind went back to when I was fifteen and having to cope with those first feelings of loss. How had I managed it? I was reaching out for something, anything, to help me solve my personal difficulty and dilemma and allay my fears. I wanted to be able to see some light. Then I reasoned the answer lay with me. Nobody else. Just as it had been then.

My broken leg was giving me worries that, really, were unfounded. I had to hold on to the positives: Paul Bird wanted me to stay with his team and that was flattering news. However, there were highly secret moves behind the scenes to team me up with British Superbike champion Neil Hodgson, in the GSE Ducati line-up for the World Superbike championship for 2001.

There was a lot of secrecy surrounding the switch, but I can reveal now that I instigated the first moves. I went to Donington Park to watch the final round of the British Superbike championship, still out of action and on crutches, at the invitation of Honda who wanted a meeting with me to discuss my future. I looked a wreck. I was really skinny and not in very good shape at all. Anybody not knowing me and looking at me in that parlous state wouldn't have thought for one second that I was worth employing. I looked about as strong as watered milk.

Paul Bird took me on one side in our hospitality unit and said, 'Right, we've got factory Hondas for next year – SP-2s. The business . . .'

My answer was, 'That's fantastic news.'

I meant it. The SP-1s had been a problem, good handlers, but with incredibly low power and far too slow compared, say, to Hodgson's Ducati, to make any real impact. And to move up onto a bike that could give me a solid chance of taking the British Superbike championship was a tempting offer.

However, I had heard a whisper that Darrell Healey was planning to take his GSE team into World Superbikes – and I had done a cheeky thing. I rang him at home from the Donington Park paddock and asked him if I could test for the team or, better still, be Neil Hodgson's team-mate. He said, sorry, the position had gone. I did not know who had got the ride – I didn't ask, and he never revealed the guy's name, but it was a big disappointment. I just explained that I wanted him to know I was looking for a step up to World Superbikes and his team was the top of my list. How's that for arrogance?

Anyway, inside an hour after my meeting with Paul Bird and Honda, Colin Wright, the GSE team manager I knew ever so slightly, called me on my mobile and asked, 'What are you up to?'

'Just walking round the paddock,' I answered.

And he said, 'Can I have a quick chat with you? Come on down to our place.'

I hobbled as fast through the crowded paddock as I could on my crutches, then dropped them and ran the rest of the way trying to remain cool and looking unperturbed. The team was in high spirits celebrating Hodgson's championship win. He was, shall we say, merry on champagne, grinning like an idiot, and still in his leathers. The whole team were whooping it up. It was an infectious atmosphere, and I was caught up in it now, thinking I'd just been invited to help empty a glass or two.

Colin sat me down in a quieter corner of the party and, after the polite exchanges of 'How are you?' and 'What are your plans?', he shoved a piece of paper in front of me. It laid out three questions.

The first was in three parts: (1) How is your leg? (2) How are you going to recover? (3) Have you been given the all-clear to race?

The second was: Have you got a serious girlfriend?

And the third was: How much money do you want to ride in World Superbikes for our team?

To say I was staggered, particularly after the knock-back I had earlier had from the team owner Darrell Healey, is a massive understatement. And then he produced a two-year contract. Talk about shocks! I was taken aback so far I could hardly answer. And Colin just smiled. I couldn't believe that the British-based GSE outfit planned to switch up to WSB and that they had invited me to race the Ducati 996. I wanted to blurt out the news to the world, but it was suggested that I keep quiet about the plan while I still had a week to go on my Honda deal.

It was an amazing situation, especially for a nineteen-year-old finding his way in racing. I had, only a couple of hours earlier, been asked to stay with Honda, my team for four years, and I honestly wanted to be loyal to them and Paul Bird who had so generously given me such a big breakthrough chance, but when the World Superbike championship beckoned, and with proven winners like GSE and riding semi-works Ducati, I could not resist its call. I weighed up the options, the British or the World, which took me all of two seconds and said to Colin, 'I am very, very interested' – then breathlessly blurted out, with no word of a lie, 'I'll do it for nothing.'

Even though I insisted and genuinely meant it when I repeated my offer with deadly seriousness, Colin laughed and responded, 'Don't be silly. How much are you getting paid by Honda?'

When I told him he offered, 'We'll pay you the same. No problem.'

No negotiations, no haggling, no complicated contractual ramifications. Done deal. All I had to do now was give the news to Honda and Paul Bird and the rest of the guys in what had been a superb set-up for me, and for which I was eternally grateful.

It was just about then that the man who was to become my manager came on the scene and began to play an influence in my career and my life. I had no idea that he had been working on my behalf even before I met him. Roger Burnett, bright, articulate, intelligent and with a shrewd business brain as well as a talent for promotion, was well respected in motorcycle race circles – he had been British champion, an Isle of Man TT winner and a Grand Prix rider with the Rothmans–Honda team in the 80s. And he was looking after Neil Hodgson's interests. Roger introduced himself to me at Cadwell Park, the scene of the pre-race test crash that had left me on crutches, while I was there spectating the British Superbike round I should have been racing in. He was his usual friendly self when he walked over and said, 'Hello mate, I'm Roger Burnett.'

Being sceptical and wary of anybody who was called an agent or a manager, my immediate thoughts were: Hang on a minute – this guy wants his twenty per cent or whatever and he's after me. It wasn't just Roger I was wary of, it was anybody who was doing his sort of job. Also at that time I was feeling demoralised, extremely uncomfortable and vulnerable being out of action and wobbling everywhere on a badly broken leg and worrying that my career might be over.

However, he wasn't touting for business and all he said was, 'Don't make any plans. I saw some of your rides before your crash and I was really impressed. So don't be rushing into anything because, between you and me, I am fighting your corner for you to become number-two rider to Neil Hodgson at GSE for next year. They are going to do World Superbikes.'

I couldn't believe my ears. And I have to confess I took what Roger was saying with a pinch of salt. After all, he was somebody who didn't even know me, a guy I had never met or even spoken to before. And here he was planning, he claimed, to get me the biggest break I could possibly have in WSB. People you have no connection with just don't do that sort of favour, do they? We talked for about fifteen minutes in the paddock and he cheerily walked off, leaving me aghast, saying, 'This conversation's between you and me ... all right? I will keep you posted.'

Obviously, he came up trumps. My mobile phone call to the team owner Darrell Healey from the Donington Park paddock and manager Colin Wright's decisive approach were clearly all linked to Roger's hush-hush overtures on my behalf.

I felt a duty to tell Paul Bird and Honda-UK director Bob McMillan. When I told them I said, 'Look, I've been offered this ride for WSB – and it is far too good a chance for me to reject. I feel a sense of loyalty to both you guys for everything you have done for me and for the support and encouragement you have given me but this is a fantastic opportunity that outweighs anything you could offer ... unless you can take me into World Superbikes.'

I had cherished my time at Honda and to this day I still have many friends there, but all I could see was World Superbikes. That's where all my focus pointed. I had built up some strong friendships from my World Supersport days and I felt I would be more relaxed and at home among pals in the international series than doing another British Superbike championship. The notion of competing at that level and the excitement of doing it on such a good bike alongside Neil Hodgson got to me in a big way.

At the get-together with Honda, Paul Bird had a bit of a whinge. That was acceptable and natural because he was disappointed I did not want to sign another contract with his team. Overall, I think they were astonished that out of the blue GSE, who had been backed with massive money from Internet giants INS, had offered me the World Superbike ride.

Paul and Bob were wondering: What the hell can we do to make the British Superbikes thing happen?

And all I could think of in response was: Give me a World Superbike ride and I'll be happy. But because they had only one team, they would have had to offload either the very experienced Aaron Slight or Colin Edwards, the American, and recruit me as the second rider and, plainly, that was not going to happen. That, with an understandable concern about my injury problems, too, would have been too huge a gamble for Honda to take.

GSE were prepared to take the chance, a risky roll of the racing dice, but they dearly wanted to bring along a young rider like me and they were content and confident that I would shake off the setbacks, physical and mental, and pay dividends for their bold investment in my potential. They had a firm number-one rider in Neil Hodgson, a man they knew would do the job they demanded of him. He was on a massive up and had become a heroic figure in the Carl Fogarty mode for British bike racer followers with his amazing wild-card-entry win against all the odds at the British World Superbike round in front of a frenzied 120,000 fans at Brands Hatch. He was their banker. I was the kid-elect. The next hope, hired for my potential. The lad they could nurture and, hopefully, have take over from Neil if he moved on.

The difference at Castrol–Honda was that they wanted both team riders to be up there all the time and, perhaps, I realised that was beyond me and the pressure might have been a little too much at that time for me to handle. GSE were happy to be patient while I found my feet among the elite of WSB. What gave me tremendous confidence in the way they operated was the fact that while other people were a little sceptical about my recovery and my readiness to take it to the limit, GSE bit the bullet and employed me even though they realised it was a massive step for both parties.

Honda told me frankly, and I appreciated their honesty, that they could not offer me the same opportunity that was being thrown at me by GSE. Sad as I was, and loyal as I felt, I had to consider my own future and take the golden opportunity, the chance of a lifetime, to ride with Hodgson – and learn how to be a champion, if ever I was blessed enough to be one, from a champion. In the end it was all done amicably with handshakes and embraces all round. Honda accepted that I had been made an offer I could not possibly refuse and that I was only doing my level and honest best to give my career a boost. In Paul Bird's eyes that was the sensible attitude for me to adopt and he was in the end totally sympathetic to my motives. That was a relief because I hate falling out with anybody.

Before I put pen to paper, Colin Wright insisted I underwent an extensive medical and he joked, 'We wanted to check we weren't buying damaged goods.' I was nervous, but the surgeon told us everything was healing perfectly and, though I may have to have the pin removed at a later date, there was nothing to worry about. I was scheduled for an intensive course of physiotherapy ahead of a planned first four-day test in Valencia, Spain, alongside Neil in mid-November when the new bikes arrived from Bologna, Italy. Meantime, well ahead of any sponsorship contract for my WSB-bound team, Darrell Healey demonstrated his willingness to put his hand in his wallet by spending £200,000 of his own cash on a new truck and some pit-lane equipment. It was all getting very serious indeed. And I was revelling in the upcoming status of being back in a world-class championship with a proven outfit that were, it seemed to me, every bit as committed as I was to making a go of it.

We were all looking forward to carrying on the great success the GSE Racing team had experienced over the last two years in Britain with successive champions Neil Hodgson and Troy Bayliss. I was twenty. I was walking on air. Well, actually, I was still on crutches with a sixteen-inch pin in my leg, but I felt amazing all the same. Can you imagine how excited I was to be tackling the world's finest Superbike stars on a factory 998? Talk

about dreams coming true. The British motorcycle press
hailed us 'The Dream Team' and I was beginning to feel
we were.

Six

IN THE LAP OF THE GODS

I was in such good company that year. I used to watch the other riders ever so carefully. I was learning from them every step of my way onto the bigger, more demanding and spotlit stage.

Joining GSE was like an extension of my apprenticeship as a racer. From day one they worked on my bad habits, encouraged and endorsed my good ones, and generally made me feel as if I was an essential part of the set-up, even though I was very much second rider to Neil. It was a new learning curve, and I was a very eager listener. OK, I had the raw talent, but GSE knew, and I certainly appreciated, that that was not enough on its own.

I was not only helped with how to get the best out of the bike and control the breathtaking new performance ranges I had to cope with, but how to handle and discipline myself both on and off the track. There were advanced techniques to be mastered, because I was taking a major step forwards with a Ducati that could either make me look a great racer or a complete fool who was well out of his depth. The real hard work would be to get me to the next level. It was polish time for the raw material and I had to shine or lose out in what was to be a fiercely contested series by some great and experienced riders. I knew it was going to be the ultimate test.

The next three years with Ducati rounded me in a way that guaranteed I was grateful for the rest of my life. They were title winners, including my partner Neil Hodgson, and the gloss and pride of that status rubbed off on everybody. Generally, among the racing fraternity and more particularly among riders, you only have acquaintances – you don't form really deep friendships. And even now, to be honest, there are perhaps only two or three people in the paddock I would ring up to socialise with – the racetrack is where I work, like any nine-to-fiver, and when the job is done I want to go home and see my mates. The exception is Neil. With other racers you maybe talk to each other passively, politely, swapping not much more than the time of day or a bit of gossip or light-hearted banter, but are always slightly on guard, not wanting to give anything away. But Neil and I, both homely Northern lads, got on straightaway without any of the sort of jealousies that can wreck team spirit, divide the garage or put team-mates into warring situations.

The first time Neil and I shared a hotel room, though, in London on our way to our first test in Valencia, we came close to ending our new-found friendship . . . and I was nearly labelled a madman.

Neil and I had been chatting and getting to know each other downstairs and I went to bed earlier than him. I don't think he realised we were meant to be sharing the room so he was a little put out to come in and find me in the only bed. There was I, the upstart new boy, occupying the big comfy bed and here was the champion, the team's treasure, having to pull out a make-do camp bed, about three-feet long, to try and get some sleep. He didn't grumble. But I had dozed off. And Neil, too, finally got to sleep. That was until about 3 a.m. when I suddenly shot bolt upright in the pitch-black room and screamed and shouted like a banshee at the top of my voice. I never warned him, because I am quite embarrassed about it, but when I was young I used to sleepwalk and scream and yell like a maniac in the middle of the night.

Neil was terrified – he said afterwards that he had nearly crapped himself. He thought we were being burgled, about to be murdered in our beds, but then he realised it was me having some sort of a nightmare. And in all the panic, I just calmly lay down again and tucked myself in without realising I had nearly given him a heart attack. He was convinced I was a complete weirdo. We never shared a room again.

Of course, afterwards he thought the episode was hilarious and he couldn't wait to tell everybody in the team around the breakfast table what happened. I got some really funny looks from then on. It just amazed me that I never woke up when that sort of thing happened; I couldn't figure out that I could wander around a room yelling my head off and not wake myself up.

Neil was a perfect example for me to follow and a huge and selfless help. His dedication, his training and his motivation to do well was another part of the all-round-rider outlook I was establishing. He had the ability to inspire the boys in the garage to do their best for him, however late into the night they had to work to do something to the bike he felt was needed, and his unstinting gratitude afterwards was yet another strength.

I was in such good company that year. Great riders such as Aaron Slight, Colin Edwards and that oddball character John Kocinski (a superb ex-Grand Prix rider, a winner with the American legend Kenny Roberts's Yamaha–Marlboro outfit and the 1997 WSB champion). There were many other guys I knew from my spell in the World Supersport series who made me feel that I was not such an outsider. I used to watch them ever so carefully and copy their best points: their characteristics, the way they talked to people, the way they reacted and handled themselves, how they were in the garage. I was feeding off them without them even knowing: I was learning from them every step of my way onto the bigger, more demanding and spotlit stage.

Aaron Slight was exceptionally friendly and welcoming, a really approachable guy, and outsiders appreciated his warm attitude. I had often listened to the general public, both the committed fans and those who were simply curious about racing without knowing too much about it or the riders. Everyone had their opinions on how they had been treated by the guys, and when I watched Slight in action with strangers it was an eye-opener. He was a hero and I never saw anybody walk away from a little chinwag with him without a feeling of admiration and gratitude for his time.

Colin Edwards, as laid-back a guy as you could wish to meet, had a wonderful no-bullshit way with him. It was his manner, not consciously developed or worked on for effect, to be open and honest to a fault – it was just the way he was. It used to get him into trouble at times because he always refused to hide what he thought. I thought he overdid the bluntness a bit on occasions, not quite as politically correct as he might have been, and I took that on board just as I had Aaron's open-hearted-ness, and I tried as much as I could to be placid, whatever the pressures, especially off the track, and not jump into controversy by shooting off my mouth without first carefully considering the outcome or embarrassment for me, the team, my sponsors or the sport. I hope that doesn't make me sound like a wimpish goody-two-shoes. Sure, I do have very strong opinions – but I realise there are times to keep them to myself.

It was as if I was reassembling myself, very consciously, with the best bits from all the people who were doing the business and had been for a good while with a great deal of success. As I worked myself up to the first test in Valencia, Spain, with a heavy fitness regime, everything started to piece itself together and I was in a perfect pre-season condition, well worth all the sweated effort.

I will always remember my debut ride, my introductory test on the Ducati. I went hard into the first corner full of confidence – and the thing reared up on me like some mighty beast. Which, really, is what it was compared with any other bike I had ever ridden with serious intent. It was about 40 bhp bigger than the Honda and, as I had shrunk to some nine and a half stone, with a couple of inches diameter in muscle lost from my thigh, I was hard-pressed to find the strength to grip with my leg and to hang on without being bucked off. I realised this was the world of Superbikes and it was serious stuff.

It took me about two months, measuring my thigh every Friday evening after sessions doing one-leg curls, to get it back to somewhere near normal. Everybody in the team was at pains to reassure me that there was no pressure on me whatsoever and that I should relax and enjoy myself. They reminded me that the principal focus, naturally because he was the champion and the strongest chance for a WSB title, was Neil. Expectations about me were muted and nobody gave me the slightest cause to worry whether or not I was performing as well as they had hoped. I would bet, though, that behind the scenes, deliberately out of my hearing, they had set parameters they wanted me to meet.

I did what they advised. I just did my own thing, building up nice and steady, and weaving myself, I hoped, into the GSE–Ducati pattern. But I knew I was being carefully watched and monitored. That much was evident after they had observed my earliest session and took in a little technique I had developed long before GSE. I went down the start/finish straight for the first time with my crew on the pit wall looking and listening. They noticed that I had this trick with the clutch where I used to keep it in, change as many gears down as I needed, then let it out after I had completed the process. All they could see was me hurtling down the straight and then shutting off to get down the box for the next corner. It sounded as if the engine had stopped – then came back on again going into the corner. It puzzled them when it happened a couple more times and they thought there was something wrong with the bike.

When I pulled into the garage they wondered what the heck I had been doing and was there something amiss with the motor. No, I said, it was just my technique. They told me I was in danger of burning out the clutch – it was a slipper and I could let it out and not worry. It was different on a Supersport machine, if you let it out between gears you were over the handlebars before you knew it. It was little alterations and discoveries like that which began to change my perceptions. Before that nobody had really bothered to mention anything about my riding style or technique.

The simple fact that I had long since learned to listen is why I passed muster at GSE. I was just like a sponge. They say you can't teach an old dog new tricks – but I was very much the new dog, the puppy, and I hungrily lapped up all the information and advice they wanted to give because I twigged that I had to learn to be better. That is one of the reasons I reckon I developed a lot quicker – because I wasn't a clever-dick know-it-all shrugging off words of wisdom from guys who were steeped in the sport and who understood the pitfalls for naive kids like me.

The 2-leg, 23-laps-each opening round of the championship was back in Valencia on the 4-kilometre circuit, a track with its 9 left-hand and 5 right-hand corners I knew so well, like most of the others, from my Supersport championship adventure. But my debut in race one was a disaster – and through no fault of my own it only lasted about ten minutes. I got caught up in a tangle with the Frenchman Ludovic Holon on lap six and ended up on my backside and out of the race. Neil was already the first retirement on lap three, so we were both fired up to make amends in the second session.

However, on the grid my ailing bike spluttered onto one cylinder just before the warm-up lap was flagged away and I had to sprint back to the garage to get the spare. In the race I had a tremendous scrap with Stephane Chambon's Suzuki and beat him to ninth place, with Neil four places ahead of me. Getting into the top ten was a target I had set myself before the race and I was well pleased with my result and, even more so, my effort to have thirteen other good runners, mostly regular campaigners, behind me. The Australian Troys, Corser and Bayliss, were first and runner-up in each leg.

I learned more in that crazy, topsy-turvy afternoon than I had done in all the tests. I had been pretty pleased to be less than two seconds off the best time at the three sessions we'd had in pre-season preparation for the start of the fourteen-race title chase. And I most certainly had it hammered home to me that this was serious stuff. I was going to have to grow up fast, or wither away in the heat of what was bound to be a relentless campaign.

Round two was set at Kyalami, in South Africa, a regular venue for motorsport racing, and it gave me a chance, albeit an unwelcome one, to showcase my fighting spirit. I earned myself a ten-second stop-go penalty for being too eager and jumping the start in race one. When I rejoined I was down in 27th place and really angry with myself. That worked well for me – because I was all fired up to get stuck in and make amends for my blunder. I fought my way back up through the field to finish fourteenth after passing the Italians Lucio Pedercini and Marco Borciani in a last lap, last gasp, blast for the line. Colin Wright purred to the press lads: 'We are all proud of James today. A lot of riders would have given up after being hit by a stop-go penalty – but he got his head down and gave it his all. We could not have asked for more from him.'

I was exhausted. I had been forced to have injections to numb the agony of ripped back muscles, which had been damaged when I took a look over my shoulder in qualifying the day before. The effects of the painkiller wore off in the frantic action of the race, and when the adrenalin stopped masking the pain, I was in a bad way – but there was no way I was going to quit. I felt so good crossing the line in fourteenth that it was worth all the pain. I had tried really hard – and the bike felt good. I was starting to get the hang of it.

I went into race two buzzing with anticipation and happy, despite the pain, that I was comfortable on the bike. But the engine blew and I had to pack up on lap nineteen when I was in tenth place and tied-up in a mega-scrap pushing for a higher spot. All in all, though, I had gained some comfort from the whole weekend. I felt as if I had arrived among the big boys and would only get better and quicker.

In Australia, at Phillip Island, right down at the bottom end of the country and not far from Melbourne, a beautiful setting with a 150,000 capacity, I managed fourteenth place in the first leg. I was relieved to be making steady progression. It was way, way behind winner Colin Edwards, who grabbed his second victory of the year, but only four places adrift of my team-mate Neil Hodgson. The second leg was a total wash-out. A monsoon flooded the track and the meeting had to be abandoned. I was left wondering what might have been.

Next stop, Japan – and the awesome Sugo circuit. I scored an eleventh place in race one – and, to my absolute joy, even got in front of the reigning world champion Colin Edwards, a real tough guy to overtake, who wasn't doing so badly defending his title in the 2001 championship with his usual level of faultless and committed riding. Not only him, but Ducati factory riders Troy Bayliss, the eventual champion, and Ruben Xaus, who finished the season sixth-placed, were behind me, too. It was hailed a 'sensational result' for me and I couldn't get the smile off my face. I was having the time of my life. I had the chance to dice with Edwards and Bayliss – and it was just fantastic.

I was getting more confident with the bike every time I raced and felt the team had found the right set-up for me. With sixteen points against my name and running twentieth in the WSB championship, I was feeling pretty pleased with myself, if a little tired after all the jet-setting worldwide.

Being away from home was tough, but I think I handled it pretty well. I know some kids of my age then who would not be able or confident enough to find their way to the nearest chippy without mummy or daddy driving them there. Stumbling from one drama to another, driving all around Europe, fourteen-hour stretches without a break – it was adding up. In a way, I felt it was an escape from all the experiences I had had in my personal life. There were times when I felt knackered, hating with a passion those exhausting, long and lonely treks down to Italy and Spain. Sometimes we'd pull over in a lay-by because I was too tired to continue and I would wake up in the early hours with nightmares, and other times, in the paddock on track, I would be haunted with flashbacks. The safety of home and my early childhood peace seemed so far away.

Maybe one of the toughest races was returning to Monza, Italy, that place of dreadfully painful memories for me. I tried to block them out of my head, but I had to retire in the first leg after four laps – and crashed (without hurting myself) in race two about two minutes after the start. Neil was forced to retire in the first leg, but blasted back into form in race two and earned seventh place, with Troy Bayliss notching a superb double to give Ducati fans something to shout about.

Then came the race I was really excited about: the British round, Donington Park, a circuit I knew well. It's my home track, just down the M1 motorway from Sheffield, and this was the sixth round with some seventy thousand fans turning up. It was good to be home. That weekend was the amazing experience I had been dreaming it might be, and I was thrilled that I could give the fans a little bit of a return for the support they were giving me, my best result so far on what was an extra-special homecoming occasion for me. I vowed I would go for glory – and I did. As hard as I could. That career-threatening crash at Cadwell Park the season before, the nine-inch pin put in my thigh in a six-hour operation, my two blood transfusions and the arduous three-month fight back to fitness and confidence to race again were all pushed to the back of my mind. I wanted to make this special.

I got an eighth place in the first race, my best result of the season so far, and even beat Troy Bayliss, the title pacemaker, in a thriller of an opener for me with the crowd right behind me all the way. I made a couple of mistakes that dragged me down the field, but I got right back on the pace and was able, satisfyingly for both me and the team, to run with the fast men into that really good finish.

I was not so happy about race two. I made a crucial mistake and ran off the track on the first corner of the opening lap and that dumped me down among the also-rans, but I put in a mammoth bid to catch up with the pack and started to carve a way through them until the bike decided it had had enough and quit on me. And that really pissed me off. I felt I could have done even better in the second leg than my eighth spot in the opener. It was another lesson learned in the art of coping with utter disappointment.

I suppose, after the best, my eighth at Donington Park, I had to suffer the worst to bring me right back down to earth. I certainly felt that setback when I got to Germany, and the brand new Lausitzring, in June. It was as miserable an afternoon as I could remember. I stopped in the opener with technical problems, then finished seventeenth, and outside the points, in the second race. I plummeted to eighteenth place in the championship after a maddeningly frustrating weekend. However, it was better news for Neil – he climbed to fifth spot with an eighth and then a brilliant second to Bayliss in the second session.

I built more confidence at Misano with its tight and twisty track with four right-hand and four left-hand corners and just over four kilometres long. It has a capacity for 75,000 noisy fans, most of them yelling quite naturally for Ducati from Bologna, just a few miles up the autostrada. And the weather was absolutely scorching, a real test of stamina and fitness. But it was no problem for me, I was getting to peak fitness and I seemed to get stronger every race.

Neil was on a mega-high after a great win at Donington Park and he was in overdrive for Misano. He snatched Superpole – and scored a sixth in the first race but only a sixteenth, behind my eighth place, in the second. I had made it home eleventh in the opener, with Italy's biking hero, works rider Pierfrancesco Chili, a regular front-runner, behind me. Even better for my confidence in the second leg, I headed star riders Troy Corser, the 1996 World champion, Chili again, and Colin Edwards, who had crashed his Castrol–Honda and got back on again. I really wanted to pass the Spaniard Ruben Xaus, a real hard rider in the crash-or-win style, on the Infostrada Ducati 996R, a better bike than mine, but he just edged me to the line by about three-tenths of a second in race one. I was elated, though. I'd had an outstanding weekend and I gushed to the press: 'To beat Corser and Chili was amazing. I just hope I can do it all again. But I really need to make better starts so that I can be consistent and finish regularly in the top ten.'

I decided that I should just concentrate on Neil, watching the way he would handle his great successes and then move on to the next race in a totally calm and collected manner. Laguna Seca was next on an arduous agenda and for that spectacular but physically demanding California circuit, I managed to get my act together. I started by giving myself a huge boost, qualifying on the second row, the best I had ever done in WSB. In the opening race I got another horrible start that left me stranded and held up behind Stephane Chambon and Regis Laconi. It knocked me out of my rhythm for the rest of the race. Despite that, I hung on in there and scored a not-too-bad tenth and then, after a rare flyer of a start, finished seventh in the second ... with that man Xaus three places behind me.

They were my best results so far. I was literally jumping for joy like a madman. So was the team. Neil was brilliant and really getting into the fray with a second and a third. We were all flying high as we packed for the long journey home, with Brands Hatch, next race up, figuring mightily in our hopes and dreams. I was bursting to get into action again at the famous amphitheatre of speed set in Kent.

For my first year in Superbikes, I needed to make Brands Hatch the ultimate race of the season. There is not a person who has been to that extra-special track who does not find it completely captivating. It stays with you long after the event – the sound in your ears and bits of dust and dirt everywhere. For me, it will always have that buzz that gives any Brit-born rider a phenomenal lift, and I felt I owed something special to the crowd, who always turn out there in massive numbers. The build-up was intense and it was impossible not to want to put on a decent show at a track I knew fairly well. All in all the event is always magical and I love the way this article in *Motorcycle News* captured it in 2001:

> From arriving early in the morning and trying to find a space of ground big enough to pitch your tent, to trying to force the pegs into solid earth then cracking open the first beer in celebration of a job well done.
>
> From sitting on the banking with a heavy heart during Superpole, when it seemed after the first two splits that Hodgson had lost pole, to seeing the orange 996 squirming onto the start-finish straight and hearing the roar of the crowd that told you he had done it.
>
> From the noise and energy of the Po Boys concert, the celebration of two Brits on pole and the beer from the Sainsbury's tent, to the smoke from a thousand barbies drifting across the fields.
>
> From the drunken and naked bloke who stumbled through the campsite as you desperately tried to locate your tent in a sea of canvas.
>
> From waking up early in the morning with a heavy head, queuing for a shower in a vain attempt to wake up and the first bacon butty to quell the hunger pangs.

From getting a seat on the start-finish straight, watching in anticipation as the grid lined up, to the heartbreak as Hodgson crossed the line first, only to be beaten by Ben Bostrum on aggregate.

From the first few laps when it looked as though he may do it in the second race to the moment Bostrum passed. From the roar of the crowd every time Hodgson came past, urging him on, with the thunder of noise, to the resignation when he was beaten again.

From the fight for it when he threw his kit into the crowd to the long walk back to the campsite and finally the journey home.

It is an experience never to be forgotten.

Brands Hatch was always going to be momentous – the place to allow the team's experience to really shine. I tried to set myself up as much as possible – we had a good setting on the bike from Friday morning, which certainly helped. However, Brands is a highly technical circuit and I struggled at first to adapt to it. I decided to build up to it slowly and I was able to improve on my times as a result.

There was a restart in race one just to test my nerves. Then, assuredly, I got up to sixth place on corrected time. In front of me were Xaus and Chambon, and the three of us were locked in a tough and interesting battle to get to the line on the last lap. I knew I could beat them to it – I had watched them carefully and I knew where I could overtake, so I settled into the race and waited for my moment. I knew if I could just hang in there, I could hold my own into Stirling's Bend and that would be it. We went through Dingle Dell, me leading the way. I was almost clear when disaster struck. Chambon crashed into me and knocked me off line and into the gravel. I don't know how, but I managed to get back on track and make it to the chequered flag. I was lucky.

From my standpoint it was a fantastic breakthrough into the top ranks: an eleventh place in the first race and it could easily have been much, much higher with a little bit of extra push. It was just a matter of a couple of seconds between me and seventh-placed Stephane Chambon. My time for the 25-lap opener around the 4.221 km circuit was 37:08.479. The Frenchman's was 37:06.005.

I was burning with anger at Chambon. He was an old rival – someone who I had clashed with before and whose reckless riding could have cost me dearly. By the time I had ridden into the garage from the cooling-down lap, celebrating and waving to the crowd who were giving me a standing ovation, the sheer joy of my result had given way to rage over the Frenchman's behaviour. It is in my character and nature that I usually take dodgy moments in my stride and write them off, mostly, as racing incidents, but when I assessed what could have happened because of his stupidity, I was really fuming. The rear of my bike was damaged from the impact and I had black marks down the side of my leathers. In my view, it was a desperate last-lap manoeuvre and there was no way through for him.

In this sport, corners come up at blisteringly high speed, often when you are jammed in among a gaggle of men who don't know how to back off for fear of losing just one place or the respect of a rival. You don't want to appear a pushover. You have to get to the corner before as many of them as you can; overtake them, one, two, three or four at a time if possible and leave them with nowhere to go under your own late, late braking. Then gas the bike until it wriggles and shakes and slides and wants to pitch you off.

Sure, there is aggressive riding and there is a fine line between what is proper and correct and acceptable and what is downright reckless and dangerous. Racers respect each other with a high regard for another guy's superior skill or a wariness of his willingness to chance it and, of course, the relative merits of the machines your rivals are riding. Trying too hard with stupidly brave moves in dodgy circumstances to compensate for the shortcomings of a motorbike is just about the most thoughtlessly dangerous attitude to carry onto the race track. I have seen it happen so often, but that in its own way demonstrates how deeply committed riders do feel about fulsome effort when the odds, even their own bikes, are stacked against them.

I cannot think of a more vivid example of this than the Irish rider Jeremy McWilliams, as brave and bold a man as you could wish to have on your machine, when his determination to do well may bridge the gulf between a bike's deficiencies and a team's ambitions for it. When the Belfastman rode for the Italian Aprilia team, the bike was lamentably uncompetitive and experimental, slow and unreliable, but it didn't stop McWilliams typically giving it every last vestige of effort. The result was that he was having to try too hard, take it too close to the edge, on a machine that gave him little or nothing back and he crashed something like thirteen times in a season. The breaks and bruises were a painful reminder that bike racers taking too many chances can, and do, get bitten. It was a tribute to his professionalism, even at 39 and then the oldest racer on the grid, that he did not tell the team where to stick their ailing Aprilia. Truth is, in not providing him with a decent bike, they were the let-down, not him.

There are times when you do get chopped up and, in the hurly-burly of racing at the speeds we go and under the unbelievable sharpness and short-stopping distance of braking, you can get caught up in somebody else's enthusiasm or lack of awareness. But that's racing and mistakes, inevitably, are going to be made – and there is little point in galloping off to a culprit's garage to punch him when he's acting clever and still wearing his helmet.

I made my feelings about Chambon known to the team and had to be taken aside in the office in the motorhome and calmed down by Colin Wright, our team manager.

He had some experience of similar situations after the clashes Neil Hodgson had with Chris Walker the previous season in the British Superbike races. Colin cooled me down and got me completely refocused on the second race. As usual, he had great advice that I could take in and use to help me to get a grip on the situation. If I could get a better start, then I wouldn't be getting tangled up in the midfield so much – I could actually be up there with the leaders.

When Bayliss came by I tried my hardest to stay with him and that helped me to improve my times and pull me more quickly away from the group behind me. At the Druids, John Reynolds had caught me up, but at least it wasn't Chambon ahead of me – that thought gave me an extra lift. Both Reynolds and I were racing at a similar pace up until the last corner where I braked really late. Reynolds had to try and get his bike to stop mid-corner, but he went in too quickly and I momentarily touched his rear tyre as I went along the outside into Clearways. Thank God that my tyres didn't stick to the tarmac. It was going to be a win-or-crash scenario. I didn't dare look sideways for fear of losing sight of my target to hit the line ahead of him. It was so close that we didn't know the outcome until we were face to face in the paddock. My time was 36:45.756 – John's was 36:45.758. It was that close a margin after 25 breathtaking laps. We congratulated each other – fair and square.

I was absolutely delighted with my performance – it was the icing on the cake. All the lads in the garage, too, were pleased with the commitment I had shown. I felt I was getting there. The way I felt about my racing, and how I was able to keep pace with some vastly experienced and quick guys on good bikes, was a heartener for me. If I was moderately content with that first race, mixed up as I was in some fairly competent and committed company, I was delighted with my performance and my result in race two. Talk about chuffed! I was grinning fit to burst inside my helmet when I crossed the line in sixth place, fractions adrift of Colin Edwards with Troy Bayliss, third, and Pierfrancesco Chili, fourth, well in sight.

Bostrum won, some seventeen seconds ahead of me, with Superpole sitter Hodgson finishing second. There was a pretty impressive list of riders that rolled home behind a very delighted me – John Reynolds, Yanagawa, Chambon, Emmett, Regis Laconi, Xaus and Troy Corser – and the crowd went crazy with excitement.

It was a heartbreaker for Neil, a double of close second places to the tough American Ducati rider Ben Bostrum. However, as some sort of compensation, a whole legion of ecstatic fans were won over by his all-out effort. Hodgy's Army was formed.

The atmosphere lingered with us as we headed into the final rounds. First off, I carried my burgeoning confidence into Germany, and a new track at Oschersleben, near Magdeburg. It has this great viewing facility with a crowd capacity of eighty thousand spread around the seven left-hand and seven right-hand corners and two fairly long straights. Xaus, with his first victory, ended Ben Bostrum's amazing run of five successes at Misano, Laguna Seca and Brands Hatch, in the third-last round of the championship in Germany. Edwards, too, was thrown a title lifeline, but as it turned out, it was just not to be for the lanky laid-back Texan.

Neil seemed to take to the place right away. He grabbed Superpole and looked odds-on for a big breakthrough, but in the races he finished seventh and tenth. It was not what he had anticipated, and way below his and the team's expectations, but enough to put him only six points behind Corser for fourth place in the championship. He was unhappy with his set-up, and a bad mistake in race two lost him three places. Even though he had given it his best shot, he had to concede it wasn't his day. It wasn't really mine, either. Certainly not in the first race when I finished tenth. In race two I was happier, although I finished lower: I challenged Neil and Corser for most of the race for tenth place, but had to be satisfied with twelfth. It was a much lower spot than I had hoped for, but I really enjoyed the dice, and more particularly getting so close to Neil for a bit of in-garage rivalry. I couldn't wait to see what our comparative quickest laps were. His fastest time in the opener was 1:28.606. Mine was 1:28.843. In the second session he clocked 1:28.688 and I managed 1:28.868.

My memorable glory day of Brands Hatch seemed far removed, but it was yet another lesson for me: every race is different and simply because you do well at one place it is no guarantee that you can repeat it next time out. However, I couldn't help feeling I was getting somewhere – this rookie was getting closer and closer to the big boys.

I was enjoying the championship even if it had got off to a sluggish start with all the mechanical problems that had hit both Neil and me, and when we got to Assen, in the north of Holland, for the penultimate round of the championship, I was revelling in every last second. It was here that the title was settled, with Bayliss hitting the jackpot and taking both races ahead of the ever-improving Xaus each time. The Aussie's perfect fifty-point haul gave him the crown with one round, Imola, still to go. Edwards faded right out of it with a third and a tenth. Neil, too, could not improve beyond two fifth places, but the pace was close and hot. Too hot for me as it turned out. I had been fifth fastest in qualifying but in the races I could only manage a tenth and an eighth – but I was pleased to be ahead of Bostrum and Chambon both times and Edwards in the second leg. And I wasn't pushing myself too close into danger zones and risking a crash.

I was thirteenth in the championship and worried – the deal drawn up before the season opened was that if I finished in the top ten I would be given a new contract. With that anxiety in mind I motored down to Imola, near the Ducati factory base, for what I prayed would not be my final fling in WSB. And what happened just when I wanted to sign off the season on as towering a high as I could manage? I fell off. In a big way.

I was locked in a fantastic battle with the Australian Stephen Martin for fifth place. But on the crucial lap twenty, with one to go, having set up the seventh-fastest time, and with a plan to pass him forming in my mind, I made a mistake and went wide, clipped a grass verge at high speed and was catapulted over the bars to land on my chest. I climbed to my feet very shakily, angry at myself but relieved I hadn't broken anything. No points. It made matters worse that I was on track for an even higher finish than my so-far-best sixth at Brands and I was utterly dejected.

There was worse to come. The doctor in the mobile clinic refused to let me take part in the second leg. I was a bit concussed and, because I had been so shaken up after the crash and the real heavy fall from the high side, he would not allow me to risk another tumble, as much as I tried to persuade him I was fit to race. That was my WSB championship finale. And I could not be sure it was not to be my last outing for GSE. After all, that pre-season conditional tenth place in the final analysis was a goner.

Aside from my own misfortune at Imola, the race turned out to be a thriller of an event, played out at a real hot pace with crashes all over the place – newly crowned champion Bayliss crashed and broke a collarbone. His bike went spinning on down the track and sideswiped Laconi out in yet another crash with two laps left. Xaus took the first-race win ahead of Corser – and Regis, in an amazing recovery, forced the Spaniard into second place in leg two.

It was rumoured that GSE were struggling to find a major backer for the team for 2002, but then came the news that they had penned a three-year contract with Ducati Corse. Colin Wright, so instrumental in my development and such an influential figure – just like Ken and Mick Corrigan before him – said, 'GSE Racing has made a successful entry into WSB. This has been recognised by the Ducati factory and we are in a position to plan for the future development of the team after the secure foundations that have been laid. Consistency is the key to this strategy and our aim is to pick up from where we have left off this season. I am confident that Neil Hodgson will be one of the main contenders for the 2002 World Superbike championship – and that James Toseland will continue to develop into the best young British prospect at this level.'

I was enthused by the news that team owner Darrell Healey, no doubt on Colin Wright's recommendation, wanted to keep me on for 2002. It was such a relief when Colin gave me the news I had not dared expect: he told me they were so impressed with my potential and my first-season results that they wanted to sign me for an extension to our deal. Their closer tie with the Ducati Corse factory meant things could only get better. Better bikes. Greater chances of success. And I was to partner Neil again. He had finished a creditable fifth in the championship and was shaping up to be the real threat we all realised, and hoped, he could be.

I was so sure that I would be able to meet the next stage of my development on the GSE Racing Ducati. My first tussles with World Superbikes had been absolutely mental and I knew I had been able to improve a lot faster than I thought I would. I couldn't wait to get into the action. The next season couldn't come quickly enough for me. Roll on, 2002 . . .

Seven

ANOTHER ONE BITES THE DUST

The bike smashed against the kerbing, split the gas tank and sent petrol streaming onto the engine; it exploded into a fireball. It took a minute for two marshals to bring the blaze under control. I struggled to my feet, thankfully uninjured, just in time to see my beloved number-one bike going up in smoke.

I just knew instinctively that I had more to give as a racer, even though the team had held back on the pressure and nobody expected me to do any better. I was feeling so secure that 2002 became all about settling down – well, a little bit at least.

I bought myself a small house, a two-up two-down in Rotherham, about fifteen minutes from Mum's place, and it became a way of escaping from it all. It was my first stab at independence – but I wasn't daft enough to be so far away from my mum's that I couldn't get back for her cooking. By now I was 21 and I had learned quite a bit about self-sufficiency, but it was still really important to me to have that strong contact with home life. The hours seemed to double as I sat in the house counting the days to the start of the season in Valencia, so I forked out £6,000 for a baby grand piano. I figured why get myself worked up by waiting endlessly when I could occupy my time with my second passion.

I had met a couple of guys while I was on holiday in Newquay. They were musicians and bike race fans and they had recognised me. They had a band called Shazoom and after we had kept in touch for a while they asked me if I'd like to join them and perform a few gigs for fun. It was just the light-hearted sort of break I needed to take my mind off bikes and I really enjoyed the experience. We did three shows: Liverpool, Coventry and another in Wales with me on keyboard and vocals.

The atmosphere at gigs is just amazing – girls in the crowd, music blaring out of the speakers, loved ones calling out requests. Our early renditions included two songs, Police's 'Every Little Thing She Does is Magic' and 'Respect' by Erasure. They're real crowd pleasers and when I shout out the chorus, it is a total de-stress and I feel on top of the world. Sure, I love the attention – it is just another addictive thrill. Funnily enough, it has been fairly well documented that my second passion is music and that I perform around twenty gigs a year outside my racing commitments, so it is always at them that I find people asking me for my autograph or to stand for photos. It's lovely mostly to be that centre of attention, when fans just stand and gawp, speechless sometimes, and at other times embarrassingly praising you as if you are a legend just because you are a world champion. I never refuse to give an autograph because the old cliché is worth remembering: it is too easy to go from hero to zero. And conceit, I believe, can accelerate a downfall quicker than a shooting star.

Oddly, the approaches I get happen more when I am playing with the band than when I am motorcycle racing. I suppose it is because at a gig you see more of me as a person rather than the anonymous leathered-up figure in a helmet I have to be when I am aboard a bike. At a bike meeting I am James Toseland, a world champion and maybe in some girls' minds unapproachable. At a show with Crash I am just another band member and far more accessible. That is not to say chances to hit it off with some really lovely ladies around the world's racetracks don't happen. I often get phone numbers on bits of paper slipped to me – and the slinkiest knickers and thongs through the post, handed to my mechanics to pass on or sent up to my hotel room. In South Africa, when I was a callow nineteen-year-old, a really curvy, lovely girl scared the life out of me. She sidled up to me outside hospitality and suddenly dropped her jeans to show me a green thong she wanted autographing – not that there was much space for a name as long as James Toseland. And it can take an awful long time to scrawl my signature in full . . .

I am quite content to be known in my own circle. To be stared at or pestered for an autograph or to pose for a picture when I am at a motorcycle race, Superbikes or otherwise, is all the attention I want. I can handle it. How somebody like David Beckham copes I cannot imagine. Don't get me wrong, the attention, particularly when it is not intrusive, is really nice and bike fans do seem to have a respectful concern for their heroes' privacy. We all know that when we are out there, roaming around the paddock for no good reason, we are fair game.

A friend of mine, who has been a great pal of football legend George Best since he was a teenager at Manchester United, cited a situation that illustrated to me the patience the really famous have to have. Just ten weeks before he had his life-saving liver operation, George was invited to Dubai by sports-mad Steve Lamprell, a millionaire, polo-playing businessman, and was a guest at a Lamprell lunch. When his distinctive Bentley pulled up outside the restaurant, it attracted the attention of a full pavement of people, many of them British holidaymakers. George, who was suffering badly from his liver complaint and who could scarcely walk without help, climbed with great difficulty and discomfort from the car into the searing heat of the midday sun and the curious crowd of onlookers, who all recognised him and reached for their cameras as he headed into the building and up the stairs.

He was caught by a woman who begged for him to have his picture taken with her husband and son. George merely shrugged and said, 'Sure, why not?' Then, still showing great discomfort from legs and feet massively swollen from his ailment, he limped on untied shoes, laces trailing, back down the stairs and into the street to pose for a picture.

Now that to me, considering George Best's world renown and how poorly he was, demonstrated that however big and important you may think you are, humility is a blessing. I guess anybody who witnessed his act of kindness that day will have great appreciation for a great man.

I couldn't let fame get the better of me in 2002 because I was quickly dragged back for the start of the season – there was so much that I had to look forward to and it took over all of my thoughts once again. Ducati did not put emphasis on any particular area of my racing and I was allowed to get on with polishing my style and improving on my previous season's results. However, I was pressuring myself: I was desperate to get onto the podium at least and was going to concentrate all my energies on obtaining that target. Everybody behind the scenes acted with great wisdom and patience. They understood that my desire for success was far more powerful than any unnecessary stress from their end. I guess they knew any more strain could have pushed me over the edge.

It was an aggressive and injury-full season from the start. I had realised pretty early on that I needed to be finishing round about sixth place in my races in order to keep the team interested in me and I was very self-conscious about my results. At race one, the season opener in Valencia in March, I only notched a twelfth. That meant the second race would be all the more important. I was doing OK until suddenly local lad Gregorio Lavilla cut across my nose and forced me into the gravel as he crashed and went down. I managed to recover from being walloped by him and got the bike home tenth, with me and Stephen Martin going hard at it right to the line. I was gutted to be kept from that sixth position because of someone else's carelessness. To his intense embarrassment, and my relief, he came off worst

in front of his home crowd. He was behaving like a fool
– really crazy driving. He blamed me; I said it was his
fault. We left it at that. I used the disappointing experience to keep my mind off the pain I was in. I had badly
gashed my left elbow and suffered concussion from a
100 mph high-side spill in free practice on Saturday, but I
wasn't going to let it keep me from my sixth-place goals.

In round two at Phillip Island in Australia, with my
confidence growing as I got more used to the bike, the
team and the way they worked, I hit some reasonable
form which lifted me after the events in Valencia. I had
two great battles with Lavilla and Chris Walker on his
Kawasaki ZX-7RR in both races – but it was the second
race that gave me the most satisfaction. The three of us
were kept back battling for seventh position. I dropped
them both off behind me, but by only fractions of a
second. It was that close ... I did the 22 laps in
35:08.589. My Valencia adversary Lavilla was eighth at
35:08.634 and Walker managed 35:08.718. The only guys
ahead of me were Neil Hodgson, fourth, and the five full
factory riders: Troy Bayliss, the double winner, Colin
Edwards in second, Ruben Xaus in third place, Ben
Bostrum fifth, and sixth man Nori Haga. I had just missed
sixth, but I was still really delighted to have headed
Lavilla and Walker, two hard riders, and I reckoned I had
learned a lot more about close racing, pacing myself and
striking for the front when it was most effective. I moved
up to ninth in the championship with an eighth place in
the opener. I was just two places away from my ideal and
knew I would keep pushing myself until I hit sixth.

As a result, I carried the lesson with me when we got to
Kyalami, South Africa, for the third round. I was well in
the top ten again and got that sixth first time out and an
eighth place, leading to my eighth overall in the championship. The sixth equalled my best ever finish. It was a
bit of a lonely race with nobody to tangle with but I was
very pleased with myself again. I was eight seconds ahead
of the next man and more than happy to leave with

eighteen championship points harvested on a bike that behaved perfectly. If we had not changed the tyre pressures for the second race – not a very bright move – I believe I would have come away with an even better overall result. My HM Plant–GSE Racing partner, Neil, was going pretty well in fifth place for the title.

Before we returned to Europe, we hit Japan and the Sugo track, where I got enough points to promote me to seventh spot overall. Neil was brilliant. He moved into third spot behind Bayliss and Edwards with a stunner of a performance to grab third place, his first podium of 2002. It was the perfect result before heading for home ground: Europe, with tracks and weather conditions we were familiar with.

Monza, the historic circuit set in the vast park outside Milan, has always seemed to give me some heart-stopping moments, one way or another. The opener was a real thriller for me. I got off to a sharp start and was expecting a do-or-die scrap with Haga until his bike packed up. With him gone, I was hellbent on hanging on to that priceless fifth place and I got my head down, rode hard, switched on the concentrated button and made sure I didn't take any unnecessary chances with the prize of my best finish on offer. It was the most amazing feeling when I crossed the line, Xaus and Lavilla behind me, and with all the team waving and yelling from the pit wall. They had barely caught their breath from cheering Neil home in second place, who was only about two-tenths adrift of Bayliss in a belter of a race, when I came into view for my biggest WSB moment so far. I was relieved and exhilarated – and so glad to be seeing some happiness in a place of such unhapppy memories. But Monza, as I know to my cost, can be a wicked place and in the second leg that Monza gremlin got the better of me.

I was buzzing inside after race one, even if I was keeping it all to myself as usual. Without being cocky, I was quietly confident that I could get an even higher placing and I was getting all the encouragement and painstaking preparation, from the manager, the mechanics and Neil, that I could wish for.

There seemed to be a never-ending time-lag between races. Once the race got under way, though, I did not have to wait too long ... until 3.43 p.m. to be precise, ten minutes after the start. I'd got off to a flyer and was up with the front-runners, bursting with good feelings about the pace, my set-up, the competition around me and how well I was coping in a mad melee of really committed riders. On lap five of eighteen, I closed on Chili, who was being black-flagged to stop because he had some sort of fluid leak, maybe oil. I don't think he saw the signals and he failed to pull off the track. My front wheel unfortunately ran over whatever treacherously slippery stuff his Ducati was tipping onto the track and down I went. I was unhurt, but the bike was going nowhere except to the garage on the back of a breakdown truck. He crashed without hurting himself a lap farther on, got back on, but had to retire eventually because of his technical problem. If he'd done that when they first flagged him to get off the track, who knows where I might have ended up. As it turned out – I was on my backside.

The only pain I suffered was the disappointment. And that was intense. But if my joy at the first-leg result was short-lived, Neil's was a burgeoning emotion: he had fired the warning shots with a magnificent Superpole performance that stamped him as a serious threat. In the championship, he climbed to third place with a second spot to Bayliss in the opening session and a fourth, just missing third place and, therefore, the podium by two-tenths from Haga's Aprilia, in the second leg. He was starting to look like the real championship contender we all knew he could be.

It was good to head off to Silverstone, home territory. I had been away for weeks, but that never stops me from being as ordinary and as down to earth as I can when I meet up with my friends. I like to keep my racing and the rest of my life as separate entities. OK, Superbike racing is glamorous and, often to my discomfort, I am regarded and fussed over as a star. I am close to my mum and my family and a lot of good friends from my school days. One's a joiner, another's a plumber and another mate is an electrician and they, together with my mum, turn up at my home races to make sure my head stays out of the clouds. I am away for such long spells, it's a treat to get back home and do the normal things lads of my age do ... chase the girls, go to the pub – not that I'm a big drinker – or to a good restaurant or, a particular favourite, out for a bit of greyhound racing. You have to make the most out of the small time you have to socialise in my profession and I am always grateful that my mates always go to efforts to work round my schedule. I often get phone calls from my mates saying they are skiving off work and telling me to put the kettle on because they are coming round.

At Silverstone that year we knew the fan base, and our motivation, would be mountainous. The May-time weather, wet and sticky, was terrible with blinding, driving rain turning the track into a skidpan and making it impossible to make full use of the bikes' power. There were crashes all over the place ... British hopes, Michael Rutter, Chris Walker and Mark Heckles on the Castrol–Honda, were among them.

It was my first wet race in World Superbikes – and what an experience. The track was covered with large pools of water – it took every scrap of skill to stay on and still try to race without taking the easy option to tour round for a safe finish. I could not bring myself to do that. In my book that would be cheating not only the people who had paid good money to stand and get drenched, but myself, too. It was edgy all right, but it was fun and a real test of commitment.

I could not, without joining the all-fall-down club, have gone any quicker. Sure, I wanted the points, but I wanted to put on as good a show as I could and still be there at the end, with no brainless heroics or stretching myself beyond my capabilities on a bike I had never ridden in a downpour. I was described as racing in a 'controlled, yet aggressive' manner and I think that is a fair summary. I had my first wet race under my belt and it had done a lot for my confidence. Although it may have looked pretty hairy out there, the HM Plant–Ducati behaved better than I could ever have expected and hoped for.

Neil ran an incredible race in the horrible conditions and earned himself a third place. It was amazing to watch because he had started from eighth on the grid and set straight to work on picking up places. Bayliss took an early lead, but even the usually ultra-surefooted Australian, the quickest lapper in both legs, went down twice in the opener. He skidded off the track, leaving Colin Edwards as the eventual winner. Neil refused to let the weather affect him – it was a great learning experience for me to see the way he made such courageous overtaking moves.

There was even more bad weather predicted for race two, but because of the unpredictable weather first time round, this was a race that came down to tactics and tyre choice. Unfortunately, Neil and I opted for a Dunlop wet tyre that seemed to have worked well for others in the first round. We went out there, struggling to find a grip, but despite the build-up of clouds . . . no rain. By the time we realised it was not going to be nearly as wet as the first race, tyre changes were no longer possible, so we just had to make what we could of it. That race must win the award for the most times I have come close to crashing in a single day. I was pushing the bike as far as I could with the wrong tyres. It was a struggle to even keep the bike upright. If we had gone for the less heavily cut Dunlops we would have been OK, but that's easy to say in hindsight. I was happy with a ninth place – Haga had had the same problems and I had managed to beat him – so I must have been doing something right.

I added up my finishing places so far – would it be enough for Ducati and HM Plant–GSE to invest their trust in me? What would happen to me for the rest of the season? How could I assure them that I was a stable rider? I have spent so many hours brooding before and after races, trying to get myself in the right mindset, wondering about how I am perceived, thinking about how I could do better. It never ceases to amaze me how much time I can spend worrying about things I can't always control.

Finally, it was announced they wanted to extend my deal and they signed me on a two-year contract to take me until the end of the 2004 season. Ducati Corse decided to keep plugging away in WSB with Neil Hodgson as a full factory rider for 2003. I was to be retained for the satellite GSE team with the promise that the machinery I was to have would be even better than my 2002 bikes. Of course, I was thrilled. And what did I do to reward their continuing faith in me? I made a crucial blunder in the next round at Misano, Italy . . .

I took an eighth place in the first leg after a blistering battle with Chris Walker on a boiling-hot June day and was moderately happy with that and feeling good about my chances of improving on it later on in the afternoon. The first-race dice saw me leading both Chris and Chili in the early stages until the Italian squeezed by and pulled clear for sixth place. That left me mixing it with Walker and desperately fending him off for what I thought was a dead-cert seventh place. But eagerness trapped me into an error at the chicane on the last lap and I overdid it, striving for too much power and acceleration. The back end came round on me in a mega-slide. I had to back off and that gave Chris his extra little bit of luck and enough room to slide through and break away into the seventh spot I thought was a banker for me.

I had qualified fifth in the Superpole and that had put me on a high for the day, but I am afraid I let it get to me. After all the buzz and excitement of the first race, I was far too eager and jumped the start for a flyer in the second. Even worse, four laps on and going well, I thought I had been black-flagged to stop so I pulled off the track. To my horror and embarrassment I had mistaken what was a stop-go penalty for the exclusion signal. It seemed to me the guy holding the board with my number on it for the stop-go gave me the impression it was a black flag. I did not want to fall foul of the officials so as soon as I saw the signal I turned off the circuit as a safety precaution. My day, and my chance to improve, were both goners. I had aimed to replicate my Superpole fifth position in the race but I was undone by my keenness to blast away to a good start.

Misano, therefore, was miserable. More of an embarrassment, really, because my own mistakes had cost me dearly. It did not leave me with too many happy memories of the place, but the new deal was in the bag and that in many ways compensated for the upsets. That, and Colin Wright's very flattering tribute when he announced the extension of my stay with his team: 'I am delighted that James is going to be around to spearhead our push for WSB honours. He is a valuable asset to our team. His talent is undeniable and his commitment has been second to none. After the superb way he has performed all season, we had no doubts whatsoever about extending his contract,' he said.

What's more, there was further welcome news: we were to be provided with the power-packed 2002 spec Ducati 998 F02 as the only official Ducati Corse satellite team.

The HM Plant–GSE outfit, without doubt the best team in the paddock, had given me such fantastic support; it was a massive boost to my progress through the ranks. I could not wait to get my hands on the new machine and I reckoned, as I said at the time, there would be only three teams likely to win races in 2003. I added, without wanting to sound arrogant, that I would be riding for one of them. It was no surprise to us because of the brilliant way he had been riding that Neil was moving on – and up – into the official factory team.

After the announcement, we moved on to America and Laguna Seca in California, where I would be defending and trying to improve on my seventh place in the title race. I had a bad start, managing to land the team with a £50,000 outlay. That was the cost of the eight-hour strip and rebuild of my bike after I had thrown it down the road and turned it into blazing wreckage in a crash in practice. I hit an oil patch at 100 mph-plus at turn ten. The bike smashed against the kerbing, split the gas tank and sent petrol streaming onto the engine; it exploded into a fireball. It took a minute for two marshals to bring the blaze under control. I struggled to my feet, thankfully uninjured, just in time to see my beloved number-one bike going up in smoke. The boys back at the garage did a fabulous job in putting it all back together again.

I got ninth in the first race after an interesting scrap with Suzuki rider Mat Mladin, four times AMA (American Motorcyclist Association) champion, and Ben Bostrum in eighth. In the second run I improved to sixth, again just behind Bostrum but well clear of Frankie Chili's seventh spot. And that was one hell of a fight. I loved every minute of it. My times were consistent, my riding I felt was strong and competitive and I wasn't overshadowed or intimidated by the much more experienced Italian favourite.

I was flying high by the time we got to Brands Hatch, even if I was a little overshadowed by Neil. He was in bumper form and grabbed all the HM Plant team glory with a double podium, second place and then third, for a rapturous response from the crowd.

I had qualified a heartening sixth on the grid, which gave me enough confidence to move swiftly and assuredly up to fourth place. I was following mine and the team's game plan of making sure I was up there with the front of the group and this meant going as fast as possible. However, suddenly I had a couple of horrible slides that made me think there was something wrong with the bike. It completely knocked my confidence. By the time I realised the bike was fine I was way back in tenth and there was not a lot more I could do to catch up again with the group in front. Once you lose the tow at a place like Brands Hatch there is no real hope of catching up.

Race two was even worse. I suffered the same problems and crashed out on lap 14 of 25. I got an awful start and was dropped off to tenth place in no time at all. Try as hard as I did I could not make up any ground. Then, just to make sure I had a thoroughly lousy finish to a bloody awful and gloomy day, I low-sided out, without getting hurt, at the entrance to Clearways. I was thankful to get into my car and head for home, 250 miles away – and a bout of sorry-for-myself piano playing. I described my double disaster to the press as 'plain old-fashioned crap', which just about summarised it.

There was better, much better, to come at Oschersleben for the eleventh round, a circuit where I had been consistently quick. I was determined to make amends for the Brands fiasco and this track was just up my street.

It was a super weekend of racing. Dry weather, not too hot. Neil grabbed Superpole and followed it up with two third places to underline his threat as a serious championship challenger. But Colin Edwards was in majestic form. He smashed the lap record and blitzed his chasers, Troy Bayliss and Neil, in the opener and then again, the same pair, in the second race. I rode home sixth and eighth, again after two close struggles with my old foe, and very fair rider, Frankie Chili. The points cemented my position as number seven in the championship. And I was particularly delighted at the way I got my result in the first leg.

I was tied up in a terrific head-to-head with Haga, the Japanese Aprilia number one, a real hard rider who would give nothing away. The idea of him willingly yielding an inch of track advantage was anathema, an unforgivable and unthinkable action to him. I passed him on lap thirteen, with fifteen still to go, but right out of our nose-to-tail and often side-by-side chase he came back at me in his usual balls-out style and regained the advantage with six laps left. I wasn't having any of that. I wasn't going to freeze in seventh place. I was too fired up to allow that to happen and no way was I going to let up and surrender what I had fought so hard to earn. I figured it had to be a desperate last-ditch, last-corner, do-or-die, crash-bang-wallop effort to get ahead of him again. And I left my braking almost, but not quite, up to the point of no return, as close to disaster as I dared take it, and put my bike underneath him to outbrake him for the crucial retaking of the ground he had stolen from me. How I got away with it I don't know – I suspect he didn't either. But I did and I heard that the commentator had said: 'That was white-knuckle stuff . . . an amazing overtaking move on the last corner.'

I gasped afterwards: 'After he pulled out a short gap, I sat back, took a deep breath and moved back onto his rear wheel. He bottomed out on the last-but-one corner and I decided to go for it. I guess it was an all-or-nothing move, but I didn't want to come back into the pits without giving it my very best shot.'

I carried that determination to succeed, whatever the risk to me, on to Assen, for the Dutch round, the penultimate showdown.

I had run home sixth in the first race, just behind Chili, and was left to fly the team flag because Neil's bike died on lap four with a rectifier problem, his first mechanical setback of the season, and he pulled out. I took it . . . nice and steady to make sure the points stayed in the bag. The second race, however, was a sizzler.

During the race, sixteen long laps, I got stuck in and found a rhythm and enjoyed the battle so much I hardly knew where I was. Then with six laps to go I saw my pit board showed 'P3' – third place – and I could not believe it. I couldn't for the life of me work out how I'd got there. I thought the team must have made a mistake about the number of laps left and not my position in the race. Still puzzled I headed for the line trying to figure out the significance of the signal. I didn't want to take anything for granted, but gradually I began to believe the intention of the message and I was telling myself, 'I'm on the podium ... I'm on the podium ... I'm on the podium. Don't do anything daft.'

Each time round, starting with five agonising laps to go, all lasting more than two agonising minutes. I stared hard at the board in utter disbelief. P3 + 5, P3 + 4.7, P3 + 4.5. Who the hell was coming up behind me? And I was praying ... please, don't let them speed up and catch me.

When I crossed the line safely in third place, I looked behind to see who my relentless chaser was. It was Neil Hodgson. I was astonished. But he rode up alongside on the slowing-down lap and grabbed my arm in a genuine and heartfelt congratulatory gesture. He could see I was breaking up with the emotion of it all and, decent guy that he is, he screamed into my helmet: 'Enjoy every moment, mate, you deserve it.'

Then we stopped together and did a celebratory show-off burn-out side by side for the crowd. He followed up by parking the bike and giving me a mighty bear hug as I stood with tears streaming down my face. The lads in the team beamed with delight and I ached from the back-slaps they piled on me.

Suddenly, in one glorious moment of realisation that I had achieved something extra special, all the sacrifices, the hurt, the abject disappointments, the pain of breaks and bruises and the hospitalisations, were all worthwhile. This, I believed, was the first inkling that, after all those setbacks, my life and my career were coming together, and my racing was starting to go the way it was always planned to be. It had been a long, rocky road but at long last the signs of success were starting to show and all the effort put behind me by the team was paying off. When I climbed onto the podium and stood alongside Colin and Frankie, I felt that nothing in my young life (all 21 years of it) could compare with the pride I felt. I knew I would never forget it. I will never forget the response I got from the crowd, with about 20,000 British fans cheering fit to burst when my name and placing was announced over the PA system. As soon as the shouts welled up, so did I. The emotion overcame me and I burst into tears on the podium. I couldn't help myself.

I remember gabbling to everyone, 'I'm in complete shock. I need a cold drink and a bit of peace and quiet and time on my own to let it all sink in.' I had clinched my first ever podium in World Superbikes, a third place in the second race – and I beat my team-mate Neil Hodgson into fourth place to do it. He was as overjoyed for me as I was for myself – and that's saying something. Whatever had gone before in my career could not match the towering jubilation and heightened sense of achievement I felt when I stood on the podium alongside Colin Edwards, the winner, and Frankie Chili, who was runner-up and who had bettered me by only about three seconds.

In the melee of celebrations that became a blur afterwards, I was sad that neither my mum nor any of my family could be there to party with me. I dedicated the result to Mum, anyway, in her absence. However, I did have at least one reminder of home. I had arranged tickets for my best pal right from infant-school days in Sheffield, Matthew Hill, and he turned up for the after-race jolly. It was lovely to have that connection with home being so far away on my best-ever day – eight minutes past four on 8 September 2002 – on a bike.

The mystery of how I found myself in third place with six laps left was solved by Neil. He told me that he and Haga had been locked in a close-fought battle with him just ahead, but Nori outbraked himself and rammed the back of Hodgy's bike hard. They did not fall down, but the impact forced them both off the track as they struggled to stay upright in the gravel trap. That went on in front of me, but somehow I missed everything. I knew somebody had gone off but didn't realise who it was, I was so confused. Haga finished sixth with Neil fourth, harvesting him enough points to keep safe his third place in the championship.

In the press conference after the race, my ex-Castrol–Honda team-mate, Colin Edwards, almost brushed aside questions about himself and his great victory to say a few more nice words about my performance: 'James deserved that podium place so much. He has ridden so well over the last couple of years and that result was just the impetus he needs to move himself up to the next level. For James the most important thing now is for him to take the next mental step ... to believe that he deserves to be up there every weekend. And not be surprised when he does it.'

He finished with, 'I want to congratulate James for all his hard work.'

Carl Fogarty added his congratulations to those that were teeming around me. 'A rider's first podium is always special and it will be something James will never forget. What it will do is give him a taste for the podium and, no doubt, it does make you ride faster and harder. He is one of the most promising riders we have and he will be world champion within the next five years.'

What with Neil's sincere reaction, Foggy's praise, Colin Edwards's kind remarks, the whole team's unbridled response and the crowd's appreciation of my efforts, I was on a mega-high. I looked at the results sheet pinned up on the wall of our hospitality unit afterwards and saw there, listed behind mine, some great racing names ... Hodgson, Ben Bostrum, Haga and Chris Walker. I noted the times in the final reckoning: Edwards had logged 32:59.881 for the sixteen laps. Chili was on 33:07.387 against my time of 33:10.923, with Neil clocked at 33:17.971. My fastest lap, an indicator of my effort, was 2:03.579 compared with Colin's 2:02.657 and Frankie's 2:02.945. Overall, not bad for somebody trying to find his way in the Superbike world. And I vowed on the spot: I just want to better my results with every race – I want to improve as a rider and be a winner. It would be difficult to follow what I did at Assen, but I was going to keep pushing myself to the limit. I knew exactly then, in that very special moment, that my ultimate dream was to be World Superbike champion. And I was sure I would be. I promised myself, until I wear that crown, I will keep chipping away at my dream.

Colin Wright and the team could see how much I ached to be a winner and that's why they supported me so strongly and so loyally; they knew I was ready, willing and able to pile pressure onto myself to come good. In any team, when the rider shows that eagerness to do well, everyone rallies round to do their utmost to try and make it work for them. When that happens, there is this amazing atmosphere and energy within the team and a strong sense that something special is about to happen. The future was looking very good indeed.

I arrived home in Yorkshire, looking forward to seeing Mum's face and the pride I was sure she would be displaying. The first thing I saw was a massive banner, made out of my old bed sheet, pinned to the garage door: 'CONGRATULATIONS'.

I wanted to give her more reason to dig out the banner in 2003 – and I set my sights on a dramatic climb up the WSB ladder.

Eight

KIND OF MAGIC

There was no holding me back. Neil's egg was about to be cracked. It was a power I had never experienced before and it was heightened by the fact that Neil had been trying hard to pass me. My dream was about to come true . . .

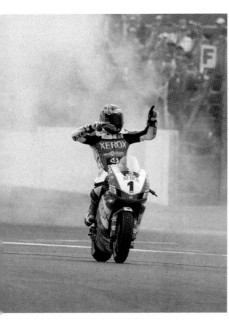

Left
Racing as No. 1
Ducati at Silverstone
2005: my first win in
the UK for eight
years and my first
World Championship
win in the UK ever.
(Double Red)

Below left
Christmas present or
premonition? At my
gran's house, aged 3.

Below right
Aged nine, at Kiveton
Park Sheffield with
my first proper bike –
a second-hand TY80
Yamaha.

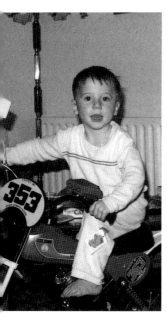

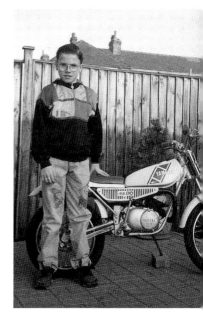

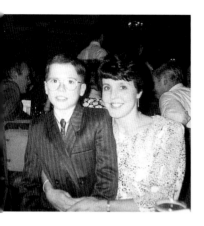

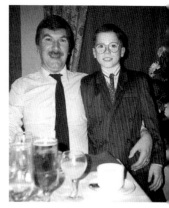

Above left
With my mum, Jane, at the East Midlands Trials Championship awards, 1992.

Above right
With Ken at the same awards.

Right
Outside my manager Mick Corrigan's house in 1997 – the big trophy belonged to Mick.

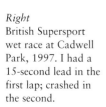

Right
British Supersport wet race at Cadwell Park, 1997. I had a 15-second lead in the first lap; crashed in the second.

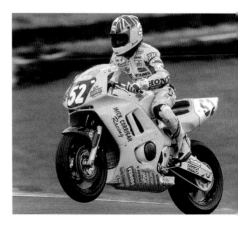

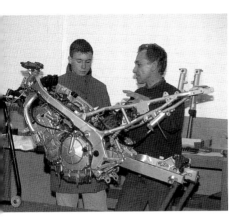

Left
Talking with
engineer at
Donington in first
year with Castrol
Honda, 1998.
(Double Red)

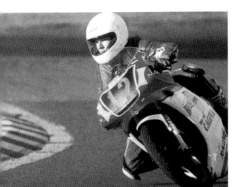

Left
A slow start in my
first year in road
racing meant I had to
win 15 races in a row
to clinch the
championship, but I
did it.

Below
Lausitzring,
Germany, 2001.
(Gold & Goose)

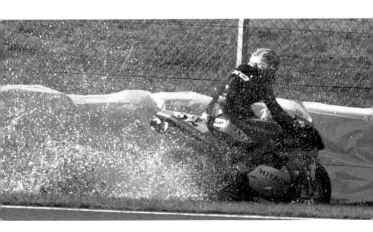

My pre-race faces through the years.

Right
1993: Racing my third bike, a Santic 80cc.

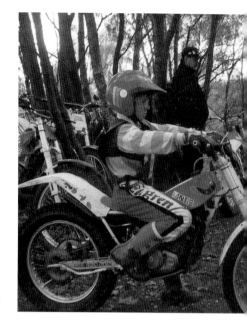

Below left
2004: Ready to go. (Double Red)

Below right
2005: Wondering if I can leave my braking even later!

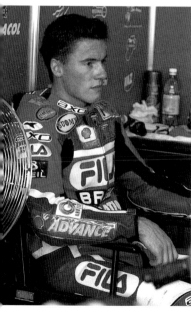

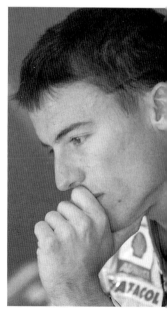

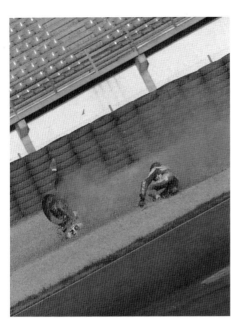

Left
Breaking my right
hand in the 2002
Valencia testing.
(Gold & Goose)

Below
Xaus in a last ditch
attempt to pass me
on the last lap, last
chicane, but I kept
2nd place behind
champion Hodgson.
Silverstone, 2003.
(Getty)

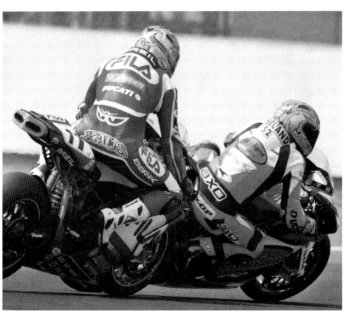

Right
Finishing 3rd behind Shayne Byrne and John Reynolds. Behind me are Walker, Xaus and No. 100 Hodgson. Brands Hatch, 2003. (Double Red)

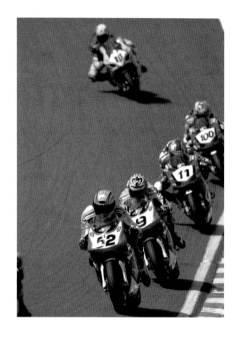

Below (*Left to right:* Hodgson, me, Walker)
In 2003, my first World Superbike win in Oschersleben Germany stopped Hodgson from winning a possible record-breaking ten wins.

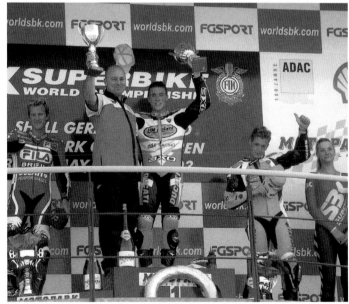

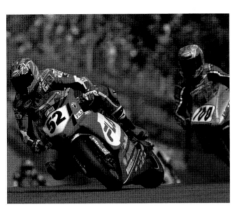

Left
Worst race of the
2004 championship. I
came 6th in the first
race; Corser knocked
me off in the second.

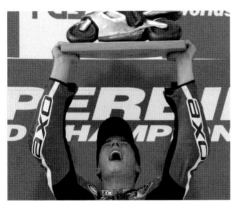

Left
World Superbike
Champion at Magny
Cours, 2004!!! (Getty)

Bottom
Holding the trophy at
Magny Cours with
my family: (*left to
right*) brother Simon,
brother's fiancée
Kirsty, Mum, Uncle
Michael, Auntie Jane
and nephew Bailey.

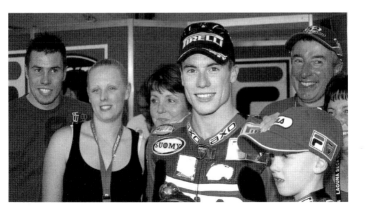

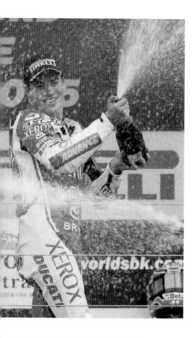

Left
First podium win of
2005 at Silverstone.
(Getty)

Below left
Enjoying the glamour
of it all.

Below right
Things are going
well. (Getty)

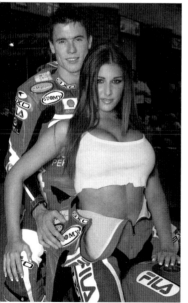

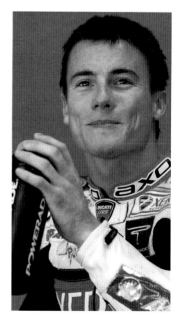

I finished the 2002 season with a handy double-six at Imola – and we had a party in the HM Plant–Ducati hospitality section with me on keyboards with our band Shazoom. I made the fantastic discovery that Neil Hodgson was a tuneless earache. His celebratory singing voice – he had secured a third in the championship and I was seventh – was truly appalling, but he was happy enough.

The wait for the next series, 2003, was interminable. Neil, of course, had gone to the works team and I was left as number one, soon to be joined by Chris Walker who had finished two places behind me after a difficult year on an uncompetitive Kawasaki that really had not given him the ride his talent deserved. He was looking for an opportunity, like I was in 2000, to show what he was capable of achieving on a decent bike. It was the first year of the 999 and it had teething problems, so we were going to be on the 998, which was a well-proven and reliable product that had won the championship the year before.

My situation compared to my starter years in WSB was completely different. Suddenly, I emerged from the shadows as number two to Neil to be the lead rider with all the responsibility that went with that honour. That is what I considered it to be – an honour – and I was going to make sure, come hell or high water, that I justified my position with results. I wanted to be worthy of the massive trust the team had placed in me. Chris and I were to be on exactly the same machinery, with the same level of treatment in the team, but I was the one expected to do better in the championship. I realised it was not going to be easy.

On his day, Chris was a very talented rider, a ferocious competitor who had riled Neil, on and off the track, to the point where they could barely bring themselves to talk to each other.

Chris, who had been a frequent challenge for me in the past couple of years on a less impressive bike, was clearly going to give me a hard time on a much better, faster and more reliable machine and he had proven himself by taking second place in the British Superbike championship. I was looking forward to the challenge as much from him as I was from rival-team riders. It is an old saying in racing: the first man you have to beat is your team-mate. This was going to prove a very appropriate cliché.

In the winter we both went to Mettet, Belgium, to take part in a Supermoto race as a fun thing, and for a bit of bonding, and even though he was a talented motocross rider and doing well, while in vivid contrast I was crashing all over the place, he somehow managed to get his foot tangled up in a tyre. He did not fall off, but the tyre twisted itself around his ankle and broke it. It was a race against time for him to get fit for the pre-season testing in Valencia – but he managed it OK.

I relished going to the gym and putting myself through long spells of cardiovascular and stamina work – not too much emphasis on muscle-building because of the un-wanted and unnecessary extra mass and weight, more a matter of toning. I put in some real heavy Olympian effort to make sure I was as fit as I could be and, quite honestly, I was in better nick than I had ever been. It must have been evident to outsiders, too, because one magazine reported: 'An incredibly fit athlete, Toseland's dedication to improvement is staggering. With the progress he has made over the last season, he has gained huge respect from the paddock and media alike. Indeed, many are tipping him as a future world champion.'

Encouraging words, but, as a stark reminder that a downfall in this business can quickly follow an uplift, I had a crash at the two-day Valencia test. And it was my own fault. I was heading for the pits on a slowing-down lap when I high-sided off the bike on the exit of the fast left-right chicane on the approach to turn fifteen. My hand smashed hard into the tarmac and I gave my elbow one hell of a wallop, too. Fortunately, the local hospital gave me the all-clear – no bones broken – but there was too much swelling and discomfort to carry on with the session. Chris, now recovered from his broken ankle, completed his duties without any problems and his pace and confidence showed he was plainly getting to grips with the bike. I realised I was going to have my work cut out to beat him. That became only too evident at the first race back in Valencia, particularly in the opening leg. Chris edged me into fourth place by the narrowest of margins.

I got my revenge in the second race and reversed the positions with me third and him fourth. But there was no catching Neil. He breezed away to a super double – just to confirm his superiority with the season's first Superpole – with Ruben Xaus second both times. However, I was back on the podium and, to prove that I could live with the faster guys on the newer factory bikes, I got off to a lightning start in the opener and fronted the field for the first few laps. It was the first time I had ever done that and I cannot describe what it did for my confidence: it was the most amazing experience while it lasted. It was only to be a matter of time before Neil and Ruben got by me, but I held Chris off until I made an error that gave him just the briefest of opportunities to pass me. I downshifted one gear too many on the way into turn one and Chris dived through. It was still a heck of a chase to the line, but he rode as defensively as he could and, as I expected he would, over the closing laps he beat me to the podium by 0.03 seconds.

A year earlier I would have been happy with that result, but not in 2003 – not in the new season that could be a make-or-break chance for me. I reckoned my chances of good placings were higher because of my experience and my growing confidence that I could mix it with the best and on a proven winning Ducati. I couldn't wait for race two. But the bike had been playing up with gearbox problems and we reasoned it would be safer to use the spare. In the event, whatever doubts I may have harboured about it were soon wiped out. It was perfect . . .

I pieced together 23 consistently fast and accurate laps in the wake of Neil and Ruben on their little-bit-quicker 999s, happy from my race-one showing that I could get a podium place. By about half-distance I was sure that third place was in the bag and no way was Walker going to get by me this time. I left nothing to chance and adapted my riding style to the tyres, my position and podium potential, and the conditions. It was as close as I could get to perfection and patience without dropping off the pace. I knew I could have gone even quicker if needs be, but it was consistency, I realised, that was going to win through. It all paid off. Even so, amid all the joy I felt, I was irritated that if I had ridden the same way in race one I would have grabbed my first double podium. As the overall picture of the championship developed it was evident that the two factory 999 bikes, Neil's and Ruben's, were almost unbeatable. Even though my 998 handled better, the 999s had the advantage of better levels of grip with their Michelin tyres over our Dunlops. That was frustrating – whenever I felt I was getting closer by each race, I had no real chance of shutting the gap altogether and overtaking them.

Without my realising it – and to my increasing embarrassment because I have never enjoyed too much attention – my fame was spreading outside the circles of motorbike racing. The BBC called to ask me to feature in a television documentary *Inside Out*, showing my life outside the racetrack. My own style, after the compulsory interviews, PR and hospitality duties, is to escape the circuit as fast as I can. I am not all that comfortable swamped in the hype, I much prefer to be either on my own or with really close friends or relatives in the aftermath of a race . . . win or lose.

Sometimes the pre-race mayhem can really get to me. Because of my really high standard of fitness I don't suffer too many aches and pains or niggles after even the toughest race. Before the countdown, however, there is the surreal side of all the signing autographs, talking to sponsors, chatting to well-wishers and posing for pictures with them, getting my leathers and helmet on and psyching myself up, waiting on the grid with all the activity that goes on around the bike, listening to the hooters and the cheers and seeing the banners and flags – while all the time I am just itching to get under way. When you have come from a quiet and composed family background like mine, with not much fuss, the embarrassment can be tough to deal with. I can imagine what a trap it could be for somebody easily swayed by all the hoo-ha. My upbringing, thankfully, is the reason why it is so simple a task for me not to be affected and to shut off when I get back to my hotel room. It's a device that keeps me sane and down to earth. Believing everything people tell you about yourself and how great and smart you are and what a fabulous fellow and brilliant rider you are, is a pitfall that will never catch me out. I cannot bring myself to feed on my own fame.

When you're caught up in a blizzard of radio interviews, maybe around twenty in one day, you can answer the same questions twenty times. Under those conditions the danger is that you might sound slightly off with a new audience – say, the tenth that day – and give the totally wrong impression. Looking back now, I wonder if I have come across like that in the BBC documentary or any of

JAMES TOSELAND

my other interviews. I would never knowingly be rude and
dismissive to people who have taken the trouble, and
perhaps overcome their own shyness, to want to talk to
me. I have spent so much time from being a callow kid
with strangers that I have grown used to their attentions
and have always been well at ease with them. I can
respond to journalists as if I have known them for ten
years. I like trying to put people at ease and make them
feel comfortable in my company.

Barry Sheene was a great communicator in that sense
and people, firm fans of his or not, were enchanted by his
friendliness and warmth. They appreciated the facility he
gave them at races. Even when he was at the height of his
fame, he still had time for everybody who wanted to talk
to him or shake his hand. He used to sit on the steps of
his motorhome in the paddock after a race and allot at
least an hour to autograph-hunters, who queued patiently
for his signature or a posed picture. But if the line was still
full after his sixty minutes was up he would wait until the
very last fan had gone happily on their way. His ethos
was: 'Be nice to people when you are on the way up
because, sure as hell, you will meet them on your way
down.'

Back at the 2003 season, I was on the way up and my
interviewing technique was about to be put to the test.
When I took the long and exhausting trip down under for
round two at Phillip Island, my championship looked like
it would be a desperate-chase of front-runners Hodgson
and Xaus, while at the same time having to scrap hard
with Chris Walker, Frankie Chili, Regis Laconi and
Gregorio Lavilla, the Spanish Suzuki rider. Being in there
with the top riders was giving me an insight to the
enormity of the challenge I had to overcome if I was to be
a winner or, at least, a regular podium placeman.

In Australia I was black-flagged in race one: a side panel
on the fairing flapped loose and on lap seven of the
twenty-two I was pulled over and excluded. I was
disconsolate to say the least, but I reasoned there was

142

nothing I could have done about it and I took my disappointment on the chin – I had no choice. It fired me up to do well in race two – and that triggered a tremendous scrap between me, Walker and Lavilla that went down to the last lap and the last corner of the 4.445 km circuit. Neil and Xaus, as was to become usual, had clinched their expected one–two finish. Chili and Laconi followed them home third and fourth. But the real spectacular tussle was ours – for the fifth spot.

Walker, Lavilla and I roared out of the last corner, sliding side by side onto the Gardner Straight, striving to find as much power as was sensible without falling off and throwing away the points. Suddenly, it was between me and Chris, with Lavilla failing to out-drag us to the flag. I inched ahead for a photo-finish place five.

I studied the figures in the motorhome as an indicator of how close I was getting to the main men, the more experienced guys and the faster bikes. In that thriller of a second race, winner Neil's fastest lap was 1:34.046 against Xaus's 1:33.813, with Chili on 1:34.182, Laconi 1:34.098, me at 1:34.248, Walker on 1:34.148 and Lavilla with 1:33.925. I was getting there.

I was a bit brash in my interview afterwards, saying: 'I have learned a lot from Neil Hodgson and I have a lot of respect for him both as a man and as a rider. He has a great chance of winning the title – but I want to spoil his party.'

It was no more and no less than he would have expected me to say and I'm sure he would have felt the same if our situations had been reversed. And I knew full well that Neil was imperiously racing away in the hunt for the WSB crown.

In Japan, at Sugo, for round three, I scored another podium third place in race one, held onto my fourth place in the championship and cracked on for Monza, happy, and getting happier, that I was definitely a win waiting to happen. In that atmospheric parkland track just outside Milan I set an early pace in qualifying by clocking the quickest time to take provisional pole; Neil, who had won all six races so far, could only manage third quickest in the session. In the race, I was fourth in the opener and fifth in the follow-up, with Neil logging his customary double, ahead of Laconi first time out, then Lavilla.

However, my big, BIG moment was yet to come. I jetted to Berlin en route for the drive to Oschersleben, not my favourite circuit, but with my usual level of confidence that I would do well. Dunlop had brought a new tyre especially for the track. It was a beauty, like nothing I had ever ridden on – and ever have ridden on, even right up until today. It was unbelievable. From lap 1 in the second race to the last of 28 long laps there was only 0.2 seconds splitting all my times. And with the bike working so perfectly, with a grip level so gluey and positive, it gave me massive confidence to exploit my ability to the full. I felt on peak form with all the other essential ingredients coming so nicely together, and I was certain I was going to be a serious contender around the track's fourteen corners, seven rights, seven lefts, that presented such a stiff, but interesting, challenge.

I will never forget the outcome and the precise timing of my breakthrough into the real big time: 4.15 p.m., 1 June 2003.

First I had to get through the anguish and anger of race one. As I went into the first turn on lap one, I was pushed into the gravel – Lavilla had overcooked it – and I thought that was it. How could I possibly get back after that? It was impossible to pass even the slowest of riders racing that day and I would have to come up with something special. I gritted my teeth and fought back as hard as I could, annoyed that Lavilla had cocked up his braking, overshot and rammed me sideways on. When I came out of the corner I was in last place, even behind the pace car, and so the pursuit began. I got back on track, fired up to make up for Lavilla's clanger that had knocked me off my stride, and felt I had nothing to lose if I went for it big-time. Before I knew it, I was passing riders – the bike and the tyres were working so well it helped me get back up – and somehow caught up to the battle for third place, where my team-mate Chris was battling with Laconi. It was incredible! I was surprised at how quickly I got my concentration and my focus back – and even more surprised to see the lead group coming back to me so fast. I had carved my way through the field and dropped in, albeit twelve seconds adrift, behind Neil, who won his ninth consecutive race and equalled Colin Edwards's record, and second-placed Chili.

Into the second race, I felt like my body had been taken over – I was unstoppable. I think that overcoming odds which were suddenly stacked against me because of Lavilla's mistake, and the fact that I now had to fight, set me up to do even better in race two. There was no holding me back. Neil's egg was about to be cracked. I had not had a race win for five years and that was back when I was with Mick Corrigan's team. It was a power I had never experienced before and it was heightened by the fact that Neil had been trying hard to pass me.

I had started well and was leading the race, but Neil came flying by. And it was between me and him at the front from then on. I attacked the chicane and he passed me, but I figured he would have to go wide on the exit so I could get underneath him to retake the lead. At the next corner he was on the inside; it was a left snaking into a right and we both aimed for the same side of the track to get to the next bend, a natural line, but we collided. I knew in the heat of the tussle and with the line I was taking that he was somewhere pretty close, even if I couldn't see him or dare snatch a glance to check his whereabouts, and as neither of us was prepared to back off and let the other guy go through, we cracked into one another. We were both upright and saw each other at the last split second so were able to pick the bikes up – and fortunately got away with it.

I got out of the corner ahead of him and there wasn't time in the fray to wave or nod an acknowledgement or acceptance of the situation that could have tipped us both in the dirt. I guess we both understood it was nothing more than a racing incident and got on with the job. Anyway, by then the adrenalin was rushing through me like a flood tide. It was the first time I had fronted a WSB race and I wasn't going to let go what I had fought so fiercely to earn by offering a friendly wave that could have ruined my rhythm and handed the advantage back to Neil. The last thought in my head was to apologise for what was just an accidental coming-together. My dream was about to come true . . .

The crash on the second lap had taken half of Neil's fairing off, but that did not stop him coming back at me as I reckoned he would. I pulled out about three seconds after the crash – he dragged me back to a one-second lead, then half a second, before I really got in the swing of things and romped away to a seven-and-half-second win. That was mainly down to the excellence and reliability of the Dunlop tyres – they were almost as good at the end of what was a really tough race as they had been from lights-out. That and, I have to be honest, my sweated effort, fitness and form on what was a thirty-degree boiler of an afternoon. When I was heading for the win so many things were rushing though my mind – what I had been through so far in the season, how pleased my mum would be, etc. I tried to concentrate on what was happening so I could take it all in, but it was such an overwhelming feeling.

On the slowing-down lap, Neil caught up with me, lifted his visor and shouted across, 'You deserved that.' I realised he would be upset about losing because he really wanted to make it ten in a row and beat Edwards's record. Ducati, too, wanted the mark – but Neil was man, and friend, enough to swallow his own deep disappointment to congratulate me. And I appreciated that as much as any of the welter of back-slapping that greeted me in the paddock and followed me right through our celebrations in hospitality.

I could not wait to study the figures – they were becoming a countdown on my quality as a racer. The fastest lap times in race 1 showed that Neil clocked 1:27.982. Chili, aboard the Ducati 998RS, did 1:27.972 and my best was 1:28.213, with Laconi on 1:28.581 and my partner Chris Walker fifth with a fastest lap of 1:28.961. Race-2 figures showed that I won from Neil with 7.416 seconds to spare and timed a quickest lap of 1:28.009 compared with his flyer, trying to catch me, of 1:27.734, with Walker, at 1:28.432 third and more than 15 seconds behind me at the glorious end.

Under the big white-on-black banner headline 'JAMES THE FIRST!', motorbike race reporter Paul Rickett captured my account of my personal red-letter day. I said, 'If that's what it feels like to win, then I want some more ... It has been amazing. And I am really pleased to have got the win. Beating Neil makes the victory even more valuable. I want to dedicate this win to my mum, and my family, because without all their love and support I wouldn't be here.'

As is my way, doing my best to avoid the continuing fuss but not wanting to be so rude as to hide away altogether, I sat in a quiet corner of hospitality to gather my thoughts and revel in the race without gloating or being smug, despite the constant smile on my face. I had not only won, I had cleared off to a huge seven-second lead over Neil at the finish. So there was nothing lucky about it, I reasoned to myself, I had been a convincing winner. That was a mega-bonus.

I reflected on my unforgettable winning race that had been almost a blur of action right from the off: the one regret I had was that I had rubbed salt in Neil's wounds by robbing him of the record number of straight wins. But if he felt miffed about it, or angry, he didn't show it. He was fulsome in his praise, and genuinely so. Even though outsiders may have thought our crash-bang-wallop moment was going to wreck our friendship, it was nothing of the sort. We both regarded our near-miss as a racing incident. Pure and simple. And there was no nasty aftertaste.

The BBC had discovered that John Jones, HM Plant–Ducati's backer, had tempted me into a win with the promise that he would buy me a piano when – not IF, you'll note – I had my first WSB triumph. And when I crossed the line the TV commentator hailed my victory: 'James Toseland ... the youngest-ever World Superbike winner ... has just won a piano.'

At the start of the season I'd had a bad race and John Jones, the team's main sponsor and quite a well-off businessman who imports excavators, joined me sitting in hospitality where I was watching an Elton John DVD, with him playing the piano in concert. He asked me, 'Is that a nice piano, a really good one?'

I told him it was a beauty, just the one I would love to have for myself. It was a six-foot Yamaha grand. John Jones knew all about my interest in music, particularly the piano and the level I was at. In the middle of our conversation he said, 'When you win your first Superbike race I will buy you one of those.' I was staggered – and a bit sceptical. I thought he was having me on because I reckoned they cost about £45,000 and that would be one hell of a bonus.

I didn't really think too much about the promise, but as the season progressed and I got closer and closer to Neil and Ruben, John mentioned it again by saying with a big smile, 'I can feel a piano coming on.' And suddenly I sensed he was not joking after all.

After the win we went to get the Yamaha. The BBC knew about John's rather expensive incentive for me to be a winner and came along to film my visit to the music shop for their show trailing the next round of the championship at Silverstone. I was featured on TV, yet again to my embarrassment, but it was all useful publicity for HM Plant and I guess it was a small return for John Jones's backing. Only two very up-market and exclusive shops in the country sell the sort of piano I wanted, and when I went into one of them in London I was like the proverbial kid in the sweet shop. The salesman asked me what I was looking for and I said a hand-made nine-foot grand. He said he had four, all hand-made, all with a subtly different sound, so why didn't I play all of them before I made my decision. I was comfortable with that, though a bit nervous at first, trying out the instrument in front of the shop pianist, but I got on with it downstairs, away from John. There was a salesgirl there who wanted to show me a special, artistically hand-painted one that had been commissioned for some famous somebody or other. I didn't fancy that. But by then I had made up my mind on the one that suited me and sounded perfect – the nicest one, she said, in the store. She congratulated me on my astute choice – a Steinway. Then it began to dawn on me that I suspected I had settled for a little more than I had been originally offered. She asked me how much I thought the piano would cost and I guessed £49,000 to cover myself.

She smiled sweetly and inquired, 'Are you paying for it, sir? The price is eighty-three thousand pounds.'

Eighty-three thousand! I was gobsmacked and went from this polite pianist trying to make a good-mannered and gentlemanly impression to a shocked foul-mouthed let-down.

'You must be fucking joking!' I blurted.

She insisted she wasn't.

John, as good as his word at the start of the season, could see the evident joy and appreciation on my face, despite my embarrassment at the price tag, and he happily signed the cheque for this most impressive of pianos. Trouble was, it was far too large for the two-bedroom apartment I had at the time – so it went into store for a year while I had a big enough house built for it. Twelve months on, as soon as I could move into my new place in Dinnington, near Sheffield, a massive truck arrived with my treasured Steinway. It was huge and gorgeous and I was as pleased as punch. Of course, when I moved to the

Isle of Man in 2005 I had the same problem with its size and grandeur, more suited to a concert platform, and I spent ages seeking out somewhere to live in Ramsey that would be big enough to house it. Fittingly, as every pride and joy deserves, it has its own room in my new flat. It is such a beautiful escape to play such an amazing instrument.

Nine

DON'T STOP ME NOW

I can't explain the immensity of the disappointment that hit me in the nightmare finale to the last-but-one round. There was nothing to do but encapsulate myself in my own little world. That is what concentration, consistency and accuracy are all about – recovering and preparing for the next thing to come your way.

After my musical interlude I set off for Silverstone, sure that I could carry on with the good work from the German round, but fully expecting Neil to exact his revenge and get back to his winning ways. I was not wrong. He was in super shape for the resumption of his WSB title takeover and scored yet another double in front of 85,000 fans. I was happy enough with another podium, a second place in race one, half a second behind Neil, after an exciting chase over the twenty laps, with Xaus right behind me but unable to get by. That really pleased me; I had split the two factory Ducatis and my belief in my own ability was getting stronger every race. It was boosted, ironically, by my own blunder at the start. I certainly did not make it easy for myself. I was far too eager and made a bad mistake by dropping the clutch too soon at the start, getting away sluggishly and dropping back to ninth place on the first lap. I told myself that if I stayed cool and got quickly into the groove I had plenty of time to get back into the race as a serious challenger for a place.

There were sections of the circuit where I was quicker even than Neil and I made up valuable time. Good, fast and experienced lads like Xaus, Laconi, Yukio Kagayama, John Reynolds, Chili, Michael Rutter and Chris Walker were strung out behind me. Not even a clip from somebody in the last chicane could shake me out of my stride and I sped under the chequered flag 0.440 seconds after Neil. I was left wondering what might have been if it had been a longer race and I'd had more time to get to grips with him. His fastest lap of 1:54.314 compared with mine of 1:54.220 gave me even more hope that with a better bike, maybe his 999F03, I could have regularly been registering much stronger results.

My family and my four-year-old nephew Bailey came to watch the race – and I carried him onto the podium with me for the celebrations after race one. In the second race, from a satisfactory sixth place on the grid, I was a bit tardy, did not get too good a start and fell back to seventh. I had to work really hard to track down the leaders. It was faster and tougher even than the opener and by the time I had got through to head the second pack at the halfway mark the front-runners, Neil, Lavilla and Xaus, had cleared off and opened up a gap too big for me to shut down however much effort I put in. I was caught up in a racing sandwich – I had to keep pushing hard enough to stay clear of my chasers without doing anything stupid and falling off and losing the sure-fire points. However, I still had to try to maintain a fast and steady pace in order to keep vaguely in touch with the leaders in case one of them made a mistake and gave me an opening to improve on my fourth place. In the end that was the way it worked out. I was fourth, three and a half seconds behind Neil who made it eleven firsts from twelve starts, and with enough points to lift me to second spot in the championship. I was still 130 short of the so-called Burnley Bullet's tally, though. It was another fantastic day for me and I had a new incentive.

With a tasty £50,000 bonus for finishing in third slot in the championship's final reckonings on offer, I was in the mood to cash in and, what's more, without wanting to sound big-headed, I was looking to be the likely lad to do it. I had no qualms about it. I had my work cut out to sustain the level of success I was managing to achieve, but I honestly had such belief in myself I was sure the money was as good as in the bank.

Just to keep me on my toes, however, my confidence got the better of me yet again. I was in Misano for the San Marino event, another sizzler of a thirty-degree day that saw me lose my second place in the title chase. Not only was I hit with a setback, but Neil, too, floundered for the first time that season. He crashed on lap one of the first race and dropped to second in race two. His partner Xaus grabbed a rare double.

During the warm-ups there was a scary incident, a biggie in the build-up to Superpole qualifying session that wrote off my first-choice bike. I had a coming-together at turn two with another guy at about 120 mph. It left me with nowhere to go and I careered crazily off the track and completely wrecked the bike. I was badly shaken but lucky to escape without a scratch. I rated it then, as I told the lads in the garage, one of the most frightening crashes I'd ever had. It took me a while to pull myself together for Superpole. But I shook off the effects, put the memory of the spill to the back of my mind, and really went for it. I made a time good enough to take provisional pole – until Neil and Frankie Chili bettered it. Still, I was third fastest for a place on the front row of the grid ahead of Sunday's two showdowns.

In race one, Neil had crashed out of the lead on lap two and I'd had to dodge round him to miss him. It gave Régis Laconi the opening he needed to pass me. I took the lead again on lap five when I drafted past the Frenchman on the start-finish straight. The race developed into a titanic clash. Xaus got me back on lap eight when he turned in the quickest circuit of the race – 1:36.158 – and that left me fighting off local hero, Chili, who had been ahead a couple of times but who unluckily high-sided on the final lap when he was desperately trying to re-pass Ruben. I was disappointed for him, but it was a gift for me and I chased Xaus home. In the end, however, he beat me by just three-quarters of a second, with Laconi, Lavilla and Walker in my wake. I was happy enough with that and looked forward to at least a repeat in race two or, maybe, going even one better for another win.

As it turned out I only made it to lap 14 of 25 when a fuel line split, a rare technical problem for our team, and I was among the non-finishers.

It had certainly been an eventful weekend. I'd had one fantastic breathtaker of a race and, in sharp contrast, one of utter misery. Costly, too – I lost my second place in the championship. Xaus, with his double victory, moved ahead of me by 23 points. I prayed that the Misano weekend would see the last of my bad luck for the season. How wrong can you be? There was Laguna Seca to overcome next and I should have known better.

California's bizarre attractions and restaurants ... the Sardine Factory, the Duck Club, the Fabulous Toots Lagoon in nearby Carmel where film star Clint Eastwood had been the mayor, the Planet Gemini and the Peter Brewpub, all beckoned, but so far as I was concerned, they did not exist. My mind was focused firmly on the countdown to the championship and no way was I going to be deflected from my resolve. Not even by the leggy, superbly shaped and tanned and willing women who seemed to be everywhere on that lazy, hazy weekend in July. The thirteenth, in fact, and that was to prove unlucky for me. Well, in part ...

In the first race, with the infamously mind-blowing 'Corkscrew' to face, a twisting, viciously downhill trap of a section and totally unique, I felt I could do well because I knew the place. I was right. I scored a third place – three seconds adrift of Neil and six seconds behind Chili with his first win of the season. And I was keeping my team-mate, Chris, a much more experienced rider, behind me. But, as the old saying goes, all good things must come to an end, and race two was the stage for another upset for me. I crashed. On lap seventeen, with eleven to go and running second, I dropped it. I got back on again, but I had to quit a couple of minutes later. And the points for that precious third place (and fifty grand) were dribbling away.

When we returned to Brands Hatch for the European round, with a massive audience as usual packed into the circuit southeast of London, my expectations were zooming: I desperately wanted to do well in front of a home crowd and so did Neil. As it turned out we were both outshone by wild-card Shane Byrne, another home-based campaigner, on my old team's Monster Mob Ducati 998F02. Twice.

I take nothing away from Byrne, then the British Superbike championship pacemaker. He was brilliant and the crowd rose to him. Here he was, this homely lad, taking on all these super, world-travelling aces, some on factory thoroughbred bikes, in the WSB show, against all the odds. He won the opener brilliantly from Neil by almost six seconds. Then he repeated his win in race two by heading John Reynolds by half a second, with me in third nearly three seconds away. Xaus and Neil were fourth and fifth behind me. Inspirationally, and to the absolute joy of an unashamedly partisan crowd, there were three Brits on the podium.

I was sixth in race one, still scoring points, but not enough for my liking. Neil had amassed 386 points. Xaus trailed him by 140 points and, with 3 rounds to go, I was third with 227 points and with 150 points still up for grabs. Shane's haul, in actuality, had not made any difference to the riders who were in contention for the WSB crown.

I was happy to concede that both Byrne and Reynolds, who made the action extremely intense, had been on super form and had ridden faultless races to overshadow all us WSB regulars. I had enjoyed the whole weekend as an amazing experience in front of a wonderfully noisy and supportive crowd who had lifted the Brit-pack riders to heights that matched their hopes and expectations. My own aims were sharpening as the season drew to a close and I was eyeing that third place as a real possibility.

I had a longish break of nearly two months before Assen, which was spectacularly, if only briefly, filled with a hair-raising flight with the Red Arrows demo-squadron from RAF Scampton, down the road from where I was living. I don't think I would ever want to do it again – those guys were phenomenal flyers and the G-forces were incredible, but I think just once up there, experiencing those aerobatic antics in the wide blue yonder, is more than enough. I much prefer Business Class.

Assen, a sell-out for Dutch motorbike race fans and a healthy contingent of British enthusiasts as usual, was a scene of mixed emotions. My good mate Neil Hodgson clinched his first WSB title with a second and a first, and that gave me and all the Ducati people a great lift. Nobody was more pleased than I was for Neil: he had been consistently brilliant, and clever, all season and his riding, at times under dire stress from his team-mate Xaus, was a pleasure to watch even from where I was sitting.

However, for me, that weekend was a big let-down. Mum was there, all kitted out in HM Plant–Ducati regalia, along with my manager, Roger Burnett, and I was anxious to put on a good show, and score some priceless points, with only two races to go in the championship. Everybody in the team, from the boss down, was as understanding as ever and nobody tried to exert any pressure on me or attempt to make me perform beyond my, or the bike's, capabilities.

I rode as well as I could for a fourth place in the first race and only just missed out on a podium. I'd qualified seventh and very quickly reeled in the pacemaking pack with some really quick laps in what developed into a tough and closely fought race. I eased past Chris Walker just before half-distance and started to hunt down Chili, always a difficult task, to move into the top three. There were three laps to go and I was on just about the same pace as Ruben and Neil up front but unable to close the gap. It was between me and Frankie. Then, on the last lap, he forced his way by me and I couldn't regain what I had lost to him in the run-in. I had to settle for fourth, about two-tenths behind him. Chris Walker was well off my pace, nearly fourteen seconds behind.

The bike's set-up was perfect and I was able to turn in consistently fast laps, but I had to admit I had got off to a snail of a start and that gave me a good deal of hard work to put in to get back on terms. I decided to ride tactically for third place and when Frankie squeezed by fair and square, I thought I still had a lap to go with enough time to have a go at getting him back. But it was not the case – and I had to settle for fourth place. I was reasonably happy with my performance once I had got into my stride, but the outcome was a major disappointment.

Once again, race two was even worse. Tyre problems wrecked my chances with, heartbreakingly, only two laps left. I had fought my way up to fourth place and was sure I could go one better than my race-one result and get onto the podium for third place and that priceless treasure of championship points. I was really up for it. I got away sixth and while Neil, Xaus and Lavilla slugged it out for the lead, I set about cutting their advantage. I caught and passed fifth-placed Laconi on lap eight, took two more circuits to get Chili for fourth spot, and sped after that podium place. However, the rear tyre began to fall apart on lap thirteen. I tried to hold my race together, but a lap later, with two to go, I had to yield to the problem as it was getting far too dangerous and, very reluctantly, I pulled into the pits.

I was naturally miffed but I reasoned that these things happened in racing, and to any rider, and the most sensible response was to forget it and look forward to the next race. That was back to Imola.

It was there that I hit an all-time low. A double zero. Two non-finishes for the first time. No points, zilch, an absolute disaster. And I was plummeting down the rankings to fourth place with only one race, France, left.

Qualifying had gone nicely and in race one I got away in fourth place and was feeling happy with the pace. Then my gear lever broke off and I was forced to quit. That was on the first lap, two minutes after the start.

I was all fired up, hungry for some sort of result and success after the debacle of the opening race. And I got off to a sizzling start in the second, no doubt fuelled as much by the anguish of missing out as I was in my ambition to climb the podium and push for those points that would carry me safely into third place. I soon found a way past Chris Walker and, by the fourth lap, I was on target for that podium in a four-way tussle. I pinched third place by forcing Laconi wide – but on lap fifteen, with six to go, I crashed in a heavy way. I survived OK with everything intact but my pride: I wanted to dig a big hole and bury myself.

I can't explain the immensity of the disappointment that hit me in that nightmare finale to the last-but-one round. There was nothing to do but encapsulate myself in my own little world. All racers have to do this – it's a remarkable knack and obsession we have. That is what concentration, consistency and accuracy are all about – recovering and preparing for the next thing to come your way.

I strive to channel all the pre-race emotion into a positive state in the build-up, and use the inevitable butterflies in my stomach as reminders that the focus and concentration levels have to be absolute. Of course, it does not work out like that every time. Varying conditions, moods, the strength and closeness of the opposition, a doubt over the bike or a dislike for the circuit could well alter your approach to any race.

You would not be human if at times you did not sense a nervous tension in anticipation of what is about to happen, especially at the phenomenal speeds, up to 200 mph, that the modern-day bikes reach in a straight line and in a stampede of riders as equally committed as you are. If you can imagine that you are driving a road-going Porsche 911 as hard as you can, you would not stand the remotest chance of holding off a blindingly quick Superbike like my Ducati. With around 200 bhp on hand it eye-poppingly blitzes in first gear to 85 mph and gets to 100 mph in about three and a half seconds. It's like a Formula One car in that it takes only an astonishing six breathtaking seconds to roar from standstill to 100 mph and back to a dead stop. And the G-forces that threaten to jumble your innards rival those that test a fighter-jet pilot's physical endurance and ability to resist a blackout.

To keep consistent laps within the race takes a tremendous amount of concentration. It is trying to achieve that unwavering regularity that seems to make us switch on an inner clock, which takes us on laps so incredibly close in split seconds of time without us even thinking about what we are doing. In one race I went from the first lap to lap twenty-eight with just three-tenths of a second separating all my lap times. If you get hold of a stopwatch and press it as quickly as you can, that takes three-tenths of a second. To go round a circuit which is, say, three or four kilometres long takes about ninety seconds, and to get to within three-tenths every lap is pretty amazing. But that is what consistency and accuracy are all about.

The mental strain of having to concentrate so hard on two forty-minute races at such relentlessly high speeds is emotionally draining and it is always difficult afterwards to wind down. You float back slowly and then all of a sudden relax and virtually collapse. You either get back to your hotel and fall asleep, sometimes in the bath, or take a cold shower to try to get back to normal again. The legacy of any race, so far as I am concerned, is one of ebbing tension and adrenalin. I always feel the need to restore some balance of normality in an atmosphere far removed from the action.

Magny-Cours was going to be my last chance not only to pocket that juicy fifty-grand bonus, but also to write my name into the reckonings for a full factory ride if, as the rumours abounded in the paddock, Neil was going to switch to MotoGp for 2004.

Farmland France in the middle-of-nowhere rural setting for the Magny-Cours circuit is probably the sleepiest place on the planet until either the Formula One cars or the motorbike racers turn up in a cavalcade of noise and spectacle. People say that it must give the sheep nightmares counting people. It is a tricky track to work on: 4.411 km with 9 left-hand corners and 11 right-handers to keep you focused in front of the 130,000 capacity crowd.

The date was 19 October 2003 and, suddenly, everything in my garden was rosy. I could not have got my weekend off to a better, more promising, beginning. I took my first Superpole – another ambition achieved – by about a hundredth of a second from Neil. That set me up for what I felt was going to be a madcap stampede. I had to make up lost ground to recapture that coveted third spot, and the knowledge that I had grabbed my first Superpole against the best was a heartener in my quest to make up the nineteen points that were crucial to a claim for third spot.

There was still a bit of bother to come. I was plagued by more, really awful, tyre problems in race one and went backwards from leading the race to fifth, just one place ahead of Régis Laconi, my main rival for the championship's third spot. In the second race the situation was that I dare not finish any lower than Laconi.

As it happened, I ran home second to Xaus – and Neil tumbled out of second place. That promoted me, vitally, to runner-up – and I clinched the third place in the championship by the merest margin of four points after twelve rounds and twenty-four eventful, sometimes disastrous, but most times delightful, races. All I needed now was to get my hands on a full-blown works bike. And then, I reckoned, I could bring reality to Carl Fogarty's prediction that I could follow him as a World Superbike champion.

Ten

UNDER PRESSURE

I know as soon as I flick my visor down I am ready to do the job. I don't have to say anything, I don't need to listen to music, say a prayer, use myself as a punchbag or cross my fingers. I am ready to summon up the energy needed to go fast for forty minutes.

Foggy's forecast that I would be world champion, and my longing to take another step forwards with a factory deal, found an alliance when Neil's rumoured switch to MotoGp came to fruition. All my secretly held apprehensions that I might be overlooked if he moved on were suddenly wiped out: I was offered a one-year contract to replace him on the fully works-backed Fila Ducati.

My 2003 season results and the final third placing in the championship seemed to have confirmed that I could carry on the battle for World Superbike glory from where Neil had left off. I felt I had done the HM Plant–Ducati team justice where I had finished – and at the same time I was happy for myself that I had performed with massive effort and determination to justify my situation.

I knew what lay ahead of me was the greatest chance yet to become the world number one. I was really looking forward to jumping into Neil's place and I felt more than ready and able to handle the pressure of being the top dog in the team. I was looking forward to all the expectations because, for the first time, I felt confident I was good enough. If I hadn't thought I was up for it, and could not do the job Fila Ducati wanted me to do, I wouldn't have wanted to do the deal. And I wouldn't have signed. I wasn't the kid in tears on the bed any more worrying and wondering what I had to do to make it. I could see a clear path ahead and, more importantly, I knew where I wanted to be. Looking back, it was as if I did not know how to quit. It was an instinct, almost a reflex response, that, from the moment I was faced with any sort of a setback, helped me to coolly assess the problem and find a way out of it.

I was growing up to enjoy a bit of mischief. The time I was with HM Plant–Ducati was superb – unforgettable and a great *craic*. The lads in the garage were capable of having a lot of fun, but deadly serious and ultra-professional when it came to the crunch. Maybe because I was so young, they all wanted to look out for me and there is no doubt in my mind that they were all instrumental in helping me grow up. You have to have complete confidence in your team so that when they send you out on a bike, you know that it has been expertly pieced together and is as safe as they could make it, even when they were up against the clock and working until the early hours. To move on from them was a real wrench, but unavoidable if I wanted to improve my chances of the title. And that was what I wanted above all else. That – or to be the new Elton John. But I opted to wait for that until after my racing career had run its course.

My whole world was snowballing: I had my prized £83,000 Steinway, my £50,000 bonus, a four-bedroomed house being built in a posh part of Sheffield and, when I wasn't jetting Club Class around the world, I was motoring about in a snazzy new BMW. Not bad for a 22-year-old whose only ever 'proper' job had been a paper round when I was at school.

Obviously with the money and sexiness surrounding the sport, there are always women on track to add to the glamorous lifestyle. I am often asked about girls and how they fit into my life. If at all. Well, of course, as a red-blooded guy in the sort of job that attracts women I am not slow to take up any opportunities that may present themselves. And they frequently do.

Success in sport seems to breed opportunity, excited women fall over themselves to be seen with the top guys and to offer them something more exotic to think about and act upon other than their job. I am not complaining, but I have always been faithful to my priorities and that means girls have always been third best after bike racing and piano playing. I give myself credit for being fair and honest and if any girl wants to go along for the ride with that philosophy of mine firmly entrenched in her mind then I am more than happy to oblige. I have never been anything other than straightforward in my dealings or relationships, however brief and fleeting, and unfailingly I let them know that while I enjoy and appreciate their company, and whatever else, my real passions do not lie with them. It is only fair.

I started taking even more of an interest in keeping fit and regularly attended my uncle's gym – he was a national body-building champion in his day. I never ever thought that the hours I pounded it out on the exercise bike or the rowing machine in painstaking effort was a moment's waste of time. I had long since realised that to get that crucial extra stamina in a demandingly hot and sweaty race, I needed to be like Formula One's Michael Schumacher, absolutely super-fit. Even at 35, Schumacher can finish the toughest race in boiling conditions and airless humidity with hardly a bead of perspiration on him. I hope I look the same when I climb off the bike after two stamina-testing races in one day.

In the fire and fury of a race, particularly at somewhere like Assen, the stress on your forearms and upper body from handling the bike, and on the inside of the thigh because you are pulling your legs onto the tank and gripping like a limpet, is really gruelling. Imagine squeezing a rubber stress ball virtually non-stop for forty minutes and you get some idea of what we are feeling when we are on the brakes and the clutch in a race. A dread we all have is that we might suffer the sort of injury that can ruin biking careers. The American, Freddie Spencer, was a magnificently skilful rider and a marvellous champion, but despite having operations to repair the damage to what I understand was extremely painful tendonitis, it proved to be the end for him. It is a condition worsened on heavy-braking tracks – when you are dropping down from flat-out high speeds to slow turns and the force you need to have to knock the bullet rate of travel off by grabbing the front brake is far more demanding than normal.

A few years ago a physio ran a comprehensive gym test on Mick Doohan, the Australian who was 500 cc champion before a bad crash ended his career. They compared the statistics of a thorough test they did on him with the reports assembled on all sorts of sportsmen – Olympic athletes, footballers, swimmers, cyclists, you name it – and the results were a revelation. He was like superman. He was fitter, with more strength and stamina and a lower heart rate, under any conditions, stressed or otherwise, than any of them and was declared one of the most supremely fit men on the planet.

When I am home I go to the gym and train just about every day, always with good old Sylvester Stallone's *Rocky* theme-music playing on my headset or blasting out of a radio. That soundtrack gives me a terrific inspirational boost and fills me with a hunger to take all the punishment I can get. I do all cardiovascular work, no weight training and muscle building because that means extra bulk and I don't need that as long as I am strong enough to be pulling and heaving the bike around and not the other way round. I spend time on the cycling machine because I can't really run, not like I used to before I broke my legs. It is too stressful on the joints that were smashed. I often push myself so hard, right to the limit, that I make myself physically sick and throw up. Not very nice, I know, but when I get going in the gym I am on some crazy mission. I strive to get my heart rate working at 170 beats per minute so that riding the motorcycle under pressure conditions becomes that much easier, because my heart is used to pumping at that speed. I work hard, too, on recovery, which helps to get my breathing right on the straights to preserve energy for a demanding series of upcoming bends. You need that to keep in the middle, or preferably at the front, of a 150 mph-plus cavalry charge of about 30 equally committed guys with nobody prepared to back off.

It's odd – if I brake late when I am overtaking and am close to the guy I intend to pass, I hold my breath. I don't know why, but it seems the natural thing to do, until I've done the job. Obviously, the other guy is trying to stay ahead and leave his braking until the last split second from disaster, but the overtaker has to take that extra risk and be bold enough to go to the point of no return. Then there's all that high-speed leaning at nearly impossible angles, knee scraping the tarmac with the back end skidding and sliding around all over the place – no wonder I hold my breath!

I heard about an Irish lad in Formula 3 who used to sit on the grid in the countdown to the start, take a guess on the time-lag to the lights going out – and not just the last couple of seconds but maybe a minute before – and hold his breath. He must have been bursting and purple in the face by the time he got going, but I suppose that's the way he dealt with the expectation in the build-up. It's like with my late-late braking, it's the anticipation of the risk that stops me breathing until the moment has passed, then I suddenly gasp and gulp for air as a release from the tension.

When it's hot, and if it is a particularly physically demanding and dehydrating race, I consciously draw breaths going down the straight as an aid to recovery and to fend off tiredness. My aim is always to finish a race feeling as fresh as I can, while giving all the effort it takes to be a winner – that way I know my fitness levels are what they should be. I see other guys totally drained, hardly able to stand and desperate to get some rest after a do-or-die set-to. They are the ones I mentally note as the riders who may start hot, but will finish struggling to hang on to the pace in the sort of humid and demanding conditions you get racing, for instance, in the Far East.

I hold a steady weight of around 75 kilograms and my height is 1.75 metres, toned but with not much muscle, even though I eat like crazy. Mum's three-course Sunday lunches have always been a feast to be relished and demolished. And it is all down to me to keep myself trim. Amazingly, none of the teams I have ever ridden for, and none that I know, unlike every Formula One outfit, has its own trainer or nutritionist. Everything is left to our own doing, it is a rider's responsibility to ensure that he keeps himself in good shape. I find that astonishing, especially when you consider our levels of commitment, the pressure put on us and the sheer professionalism demanded these days with so much money invested, for instance, in factory teams.

At Ducati, we do have fitness tests three times a year at the factory in Bologna. One before the season starts just to make sure you haven't eaten too much Christmas pud, and then a couple more times to monitor your progress – but it's all pretty lightly done. It used to be a bench press to check if you could heave your own body weight. I have always been around 70–74 kg, but I was the record-holder, which surprised them and pleased me. I could easily do eighteen repetitions of my own weight. It became a matter of personal pride, and a challenge, to beat the other guys and my own target every fresh time there. If at any time anybody equalled or bettered me, it fired me up, as any challenge always does, to outdo them. Now they make us wear a mask and put us on a bike to measure our oxygen levels and heart rate. But that's it. The only other tests are for your racing licence (eyesight and so on). The reasoning seems to be that when a team signs you, they know you must already have a certain level of fitness. If I had my way, I would make sure every team had a fitness expert and a nutritionist. It makes sense, doesn't it?

One of the more serious problems we have as racers is sometimes being too eager for our own good. I have lost count of how many times I have seen wincing, pain-wracked riders climb aboard bikes to race when they would have been more suited to doing nothing more vigorous or dangerous than plumping a pillow to lie in a hospital bed. It is in our nature to insist through firmly clenched teeth with our leg in three bits that we are OK to race when sometimes we are nowhere near fit enough even to walk. I am a prime example. When I smashed both ankles at Monza, my refusal to accept that I was nowhere near healthy enough to get back on a bike bordered on stupidity. I was seventeen – and, clearly, I needed some stern advice to bring me to my senses. I wonder if I would have accepted it.

I looked forward with growing hope that the 999, which had carried Neil to his title success, would do the same for me. I had been well jealous of Neil's bike for a long time and couldn't wait to ride it. My 998 looked about five years older and the whole package seemed far less cool. I was desperate to get into my new leathers and go prancing around asking, 'Does my bum look big in these?' The 999 was a mega-looking mean machine and, compared to my previous 998, it was a towering promise that I wouldn't have to compensate for the bike's comparative lack of speed with extra risk-taking. The team, too, knew all about winning and, as the world's number one WSB outfit, they enjoyed an expectation of even more success to come. With all these considerations it left me in no doubt that I was firmly in the frame for a glorious run for the 2004 championship. As I said in the press: 'The Fila Ducati looks mega.'

I didn't want to go around shouting my mouth off about what I was going to do, I just wanted to get on with things.

I prepared for my 2004 campaign to take up where Neil Hodgson had left off. Xaus, too, nicknamed 'The Rubberman' because of his remarkable ability to bounce right back up from the most serious of crashes, shifted across to MotoGp, much to my relief but not, I am sure, to Neil's, who had the great joy at having his erratic, long-legged partner as a Ducati team-mate for at least another year. Ruben has certainly always been spectacular – all legs and awkward angles and a frequent faller. He's not necessarily dangerous, but he has a loose riding style that always keeps him right on the edge and made me a bit wary to be around him on track and, I have to say, sceptical about his ability. Away from the circuit he was an impressively intelligent and suave guy who speaks four languages. Still, without any spite, it was a relief to see him move on.

The UK motorcycle sales market is a big deal for Ducati and that is why they were keen to have another British rider in their 2004 WSB line-up. Their profile in France, though, wasn't too good and they were struggling there, so the team opted for Régis Laconi, a Frenchman, in a bid to revitalise showroom interest in the marque. I have to say he was looking ready for a promotion to the full factory team. He had put in some consistent performances in the 2003 season and had finished fourth behind me in the championship. On a better bike than the 998 he was obviously going to be a big threat. However, I knew I could beat him and, with growing anticipation that it was going to be my breakthrough year, I warmed to the challenge. I was absolutely certain he would present a threat and I was right.

We went to Valencia for pre-season testing and, even though I set some quick times and we dominated the sessions, I found it a tough experience trying to master the 999 and its vagaries that were new to me compared with the 998. I knew it was going to be difficult, but I didn't realise it was going to be such a huge learning curve. I found the chassis and the riding style I needed to adapt completely different. But by the time testing was finished I was not far off the times I had set earlier in the year. Laconi, however, kept topping the time sheets and I was determined to alter that state of affairs when the season proper got under way.

The first race, back in Valencia, gave me my dream start. A win in the opener and a second place in the next leg. Régis was nowhere. I took an early lead in the eleven-round championship, but I'd had a near miss that reminded me I wasn't as clever as I thought I was. I fell off in free practice, in the build-up to qualifying, after losing control on the extremely dusty track. I got my act together and earned second place on the grid, beating Frankie Chili in the first leg with Chris Walker, on Foggy's Petronus, third.

I was happy enough and grinned to everybody in sight: 'There is nothing like winning.' And, oh boy, did I mean it! I was relieved to take the flag after everything that had gone on in the damp conditions: Haga, Laconi and Corser failed to finish. Nori Haga rode his luck second time out with him first and me second. He whizzed past me and then I was sure I was off when Corser crashed right next to me. I chased Nori for 23 laps and then took the sensible option and settled for second place with the points and the championship lead. It had been a nerve-wracking week-end and I was relieved to get it over and done with so rewardingly. It was a clear sign for what lay ahead. I began to realise that this championship was going to see the upfront action very close. There were going to be quite a few different winners – and hopefully some good scraps right to the end, because that's what the fans want to watch.

It's a shame the fans can't see Régis's comically oddball antics in the garage, too: an interesting and amusing spectacle to say the least. He stands wordlessly in a corner, facing the wall, helmet and gloves on, and pounds his chest like King Kong or a gorilla warning off trespassers on his territory. God only knows what he is trying to do to himself – boost his adrenalin, I guess. But he does flap about and is quite flamboyant and emotional and I have to smile to myself. We make quite a pair. I know as soon as I flick my visor down I am ready to do the job. I don't have to say anything, I don't need to listen to music, say a prayer, use myself as a punchbag or cross my fingers. I am ready to summon up the energy needed to go fast for forty minutes.

Régis's ritual worked for him in the second round in Australia. He won the opening leg and the best I could do was third – with a tumble in the second leg. It was a thriller of a speedway-style finish to the first session. I found it a hell of a job to put the power down and Steve Martin caught and passed me, but then he had the same problem. I hung onto him as best I could, made a mistake with six laps to go, but managed to get back for what was a real fighting third place. In the second race we made a slight modification to the rear-end set-up, which gave me a much better feel. Trouble was, once again, it boosted my confidence a little too much. When I hared into the Siberia turn I pushed the front too hard. There was little or no rear-end grip, anyway, and the bike got away from me. My advantage over Chili in the championship slipped to five points. I had the gut feeling it was going to get tougher, as the season developed, to take the title.

I learned what it was like to get knocked off your stride and off the top spot in Misano. Qualifying was a nightmare in the wet weather and I struggled – and failed miserably – to master the tricky conditions. I had got myself into the top ten, but then I plummeted down to a dreadfully disappointing twentieth on the grid. We fiddled about with the settings far too much. I even switched bikes in a bid to solve the problems – but I was unable to clock a decent time and all the other guys bettered my performance. Talk about being knocked down a peg or two. I couldn't remember when I was last that far back. It left me far too much ground to have to make up and, clearly, my title lead was under serious threat even before the two races had started. Laconi rubbed the salt in my very wounded pride with a win and a second while I trundled home tenth and sixth. I should have had an eighth in race one, but Lucio Pedercini fell off right in front of me and I had to take avoiding action to miss him. That let two other guys in to pass me.

In race two I rode my heart out to carve a path from twentieth on the grid to sixth place, but that was as high as I could manage without benefiting from somebody else's misfortune, and that didn't happen. I had to be happy with the points for sixth place to keep alive my chances for the crown. Chili inched ahead with 97 points to my 77, with Laconi and 2003 Supersport champion Chris Vermeulen (an Aussie and Barry Sheene's protégé) jointly on 70. I was happy with the challenge, and anyway, I had no choice. This was to be a championship earned on merit.

With this in mind, I tried to prepare myself for my return to Monza. Travelling to the track I could feel an ache in the pit of my stomach. The track has such a pull over me, such a cloud of memories, and every time I return I can't help reliving my bad crash – and the images of my team-mate, Michael Paquay, before he took to the track for the last time. This year I needed the track to be good to me more than ever – I have never felt so apprehensive and longed for my luck to change just this once.

During the opener Chris Vermeulen was extremely switched on and determined – I tussled with him to snatch second place. My head was a mess. I just couldn't feel at ease. We could not find the right way to go with the settings to improve my 'feeling' on the bike. The engineers scratched their heads and we had to study the telemetry, the sensors on the bike that electronically – and magically, to my mind – measure rev levels, wheel speed, the travel on the front forks and the behaviour of the suspension, to try and find a solution, a compromise, that made me more comfortable with the bike's behaviour. The tyres were not a problem, but I just did not feel comfortable and it was an urgent situation to get the best combination at the front and the back. It was frustrating for everybody in the team, but particularly for me because I knew I could express myself and my potential and be a winner if only we got the mix right.

Then another battle, this time with Garry McCoy in race two, put me in third place behind Vermeulen. However, at long last, there was a slice of luck for me at Monza. Chris was disqualified. His engine cut-out switch, devised, of course, to kill the motor in the event of a crash, failed to function when it was tested after the race. I earned myself two podium places, a second and a third, with Laconi securing his first ever victory double. That leapfrogged him over both Chili and me into top spot and I was hanging on in there in second place, three points adrift of my team-mate. It was just the boost I needed after the awfully costly setbacks in Misano the rainy round before.

I climbed back to the top of the WSB tree with a pair of seconds when we got to Oschersleben for a German points-fest. That was the scene of my very first Superbike win a year before, and I had even more reason to be pleased this time round because my harvest of points put me right back in the frame for the title. With just six rounds to go, the excitement was growing and the anticipation of a neck-and-neck finish looked a racing certainty. Haga and Laconi were the winners but my double gave me enough of a lift to sneak ahead of Régis by just two points. Chili was locked in third place. I was consistent now – but not a winner. And I reasoned that as long as I clinched the title it wouldn't matter whether I did it on outright wins or as a patient collector of vital podiums and the points that went with them. I was getting consistently quick and bold enough when it most mattered. And patient, too. The championship was full of ups and downs so it could not fail to be interesting. If I could not win a race, the safest option was to get as high as I could without trashing the bike in unnecessary and rash acts of bravado for the sake of it. I had nothing to prove as a racer, but a lot to show as a potential, and sensible, champion. In addition, I had got the bike working OK. That was a huge bonus.

Although I was happy with the points I was accumulating, second places were doing my head in, as they would any true-born racer who yearns to be a winner. Sure, I realised I had to be patient, understood the implications of trying too hard, and reasoned that taking the title would be worth all the disappointment of not standing on the top step of every podium every time I raced, but I was just so close and hungry for the final accomplishment. I'm glad I remained patient because, when we got to Silverstone for the British round, with 68,000 fans praying for a home triumph – a triumph I hoped would be mine – I faced another scary upset.

I had the fastest and worst crash of my life in the first race. It was at Abbey and I was doing around 150 mph even though I was struggling with the front-end grip. It was some sort of miracle that I did no more damage to myself than bang my thumb, bruise my back and crack three ribs. I was shaken and a bit banged about, but I just wanted to get back on the bike and put in a gritty performance in race two a couple of hours later. I was up for it, lifted by the fans, and determined to make amends. Then Chili came by too close and took me out. By the time I got back into the swing and tried to catch Leon Haslam my tyres started to go off again. I stuck at it and was being pulled along by the leaders, doing some useful times – only a tenth off my Superpole lap. However, it was all over before it began, really. I finished fifth and bang went my lead in the title. Laconi, who had also fallen off in race one, was top on 171 against my 168. If Régis hadn't dropped his bike he would have stretched out an advantage that would have been a crucial factor in the numbers game. Thankfully, I had not lost too much ground on him.

Laguna Seca was next. And word had obviously got round because 93,000 people crowded into the Californian circuit for what turned out to be a tingling spectacular, just the right and exciting sort of advert for World Superbikes and motorbike racing in general. It was a real treat to be part of the show – and a treat to really take on my team-mate, who was proving to be a big obstacle to my ambitions. It was my time to turn up the heat with four rounds on the schedule. And I did. Aggressively.

The first race was a complete showdown, very hard with two guys, him and me, not prepared to yield an inch. I led early on until my tyres started to play up, but still managed to get enough out of them to clinch fifth place. I followed that up with a second place in race two behind Chris Vermeulen, who notched a well-deserved double.

Race one did nothing to cement my friendship with Laconi. We had more than an altercation while battling for fourth place. We banged into each other more times than I can remember, leaned on one another and, generally, ruthlessly jousted like a pair of duelling knights. I tried to stave off the reverse effects of a tyre yet again going off and leaving me fighting like mad for enough grip not only to keep me mounted, but to keep me in the race. Every single point, with the title race being so tight, was as precious as diamonds. And neither of us was prepared to let slip any opportunity to humble the other guy – even if we did share a team and a garage.

I was quoted afterwards as saying, 'I had a real close battle with Régis which got a bit out of hand a couple of times, but we both stayed on. It was just close racing and I would bet it was good to watch.' I am not so sure he shared my opinion because there was no real love lost between us.

The boys in the garage made some slight changes to the rear setting to try to get me a little more grip, which seemed to work. Race two was another nail-biter and more of the same with Laconi, although this time with Vermeulen joining the fray to give it added spice for an extremely enthralled crowd. All credit to Chris, but the battle was very frustrating for me. When he dived under me at turn two I thought it was game over, but I got settled into a good rhythm and kept with him and, at the same time, made sure Régis stayed behind me. Chris was relentless in defence of his position and there was never the slightest opportunity for me to squeeze past. All I could do was follow him home, fretting and struggling all the way.

I retook the championship lead on 201 points with Laconi on 198. Vermeulen was third on 187 with Haga on 162 next, ahead of fifth-placed Chili on 160.

There reaches a stage in the championship when you are prepared for the see-sawing results and are just totally overpowered to put yourself in your rightful place at the top. For me, that time was round eight: Brands Hatch. It was, therefore, like being stripped of all my senses when I didn't perform well. I left the Kent circuit feeling utterly drained and lifeless, apologising for an inept and ineffectual display by both me and the bike to a vast army of fans who had demonstrated their support in the noisiest, most colourful way they could. If I could have converted their enthusiasm and loyalty into action on the track I would have been walking tall at the end of the day. As it turned out, I slumped down to fourth place in the championship after a disastrous Superpole qualifying session that left me having to struggle from twelfth place on the grid. Because I couldn't force a way through the traffic, seventh place in the first race was all I could manage.

In race two the bike suffered an oil-cooler leak after only three laps – but I got what I hoped would be a reprieve from further embarrassment when the race was stopped and I was able to switch to my back-up bike for the resumption. But it all went horribly, and painfully, wrong again just two corners later. I was wiped out, shoved into the gravel by Troy Corser on the Petronus.

It was as gloomy an afternoon of abject misery as I could remember, more especially because time was fast running out to claim that number one dream. The points for the decider were becoming more precious and hard to get by the race. I could not believe how badly things could turn out, especially when the expectations of around 100,000 people were so faithfully placed on my shoulders. Could anything be worse than disappointing yourself and your home crowd? I sat glumly in the garage moaning about my sore neck from the crash and swearing that I'd lost the championship lead for good. I had dropped to fourth and was thoroughly pissed off.

I made a public apology in a sullen tone: 'I can only apologise and say that, honestly, I have given a hundred per cent all weekend, but it hasn't worked out for me. I am sorry for everybody who turned up to see a British winner. That was down to me. So let's forget it, get it over with and move on to the next round.'

Haga had scored a win double. Laconi was second in race one, but then crashed out at Graham Hill bend in the second leg – that was a bit of a favour, thank you, Régis. However, he was back on top in the championship, this time with Vermeulen taking second place only two points behind. Haga was third, just two ahead of my tally.

If Brands Hatch was one of the lowest points of 2004, Assen was one of the highlights. I came storming back to retake the lead with only two rounds left. There was a crowd of 76,000 packed in to watch the action that seemed to take a dramatic turn at every venue. It was certainly riveting stuff that I couldn't have lifted from the script of one of my favourite action films. Fun maybe for the WSB fans, but nerve-wracking for contenders for a title that was getting increasingly tight. We were reaching the stage where something just had to give and where the coolest head or boldest heart would triumph in final glory.

How many British bikers had followed us to Assen in Northern Holland I have no idea – but there seemed to be thousands of them. They were everywhere – and it was doubly heartening to see banners supporting me despite my shock show at home. It was impossible to move about the town, drive into the circuit or walk around the paddock without well-wishers seeking me out for a handshake and a good-luck pat on the back. It lifted my morale sky-high and I determined to pay back the massive backing with all the effort I could summon up. I told myself, right, it is now or never. Crash or bust.

In the first sixteen-lapper, I hit the high spots with a win and I was flying. I won in front of Chili, with Laconi third, Haga next and Vermeulen, at last out of it, fifth. It's such a fast and flowing circuit and difficult to pull away, I only got a two-second gap in the first race. The other guys were battling behind me and slowed each other down. In the second race Vermeulen came back at me for a win, but I finished second, with Haga and Chili third and fourth and Laconi next. I could sense them behind me on every curve. I was ecstatic – such superb racing and elbow-bashing with Nori Haga and so close with Chris Vermeulen! That is what every race should be like. I hate great races where I come second – but I needed to get 45 points out of this weekend if I wanted to win the title. There were so many other talented riders who were knocking on the door of the championship, but I had to hang in there. I was back on top of the heap with only two rounds to go – Imola, my real bogey track, and Magny-Cours, Laconi's home ground – with Vermeulen three points behind me on 253 and Régis on 245. It was going to go right down to the wire.

I had suffered crashes and bizarre setbacks, like my gear lever falling off and tyres exploding, at the Italian track in the past and it was with some trepidation I arrived there wondering what other little surprises the place had in store for me. I was good and fast there, but there was that run of bad luck overshadowing any build-up of confidence; not that I am superstitious in any way, but these odd things do have a habit of repeating themselves at bad-luck tracks. As it turned out, and with a 72,000 crowd on hand, it set the stage for a nail-biter of a finale.

It was to be a three-horse race for the championship, with Vermeulen creeping into the final reckonings.

Laconi dealt with the challenge of Vermeulen in race one with me third, ahead of Haga – and later took his second win of the afternoon. That was a tremendous free-for-all, right on the edge, and right up to the flag. It got off to a spectacular start when Chris crashed out on the warm-up lap – and ended with me and Laconi mixing it at high speed and shoulder-charging each other right on the line for him to snatch a win by just four-hundredths of a second, half a wheel, in a fantastic photo finish. I got two podiums – but Laconi slipped into a four-point title lead with a double of wins.

Back in the garage I discussed Régis with the boys – he was obviously doing his best to protect his line going into the last chicane. Unfortunately, the finish line is so close to the chicane and I just had to try and win. It was a fantastic race with neither of us willing to back off. The pass he made was a tough one – but I didn't want to finish second if I had the breath and balls to avoid it, and I was determined not to. It made for a tasty finish. But he came out tops and I wished him the best of luck.

Régis and I may have been team-mates but, as I told everybody, we were heading to Magny-Cours for the finale and there would be no love lost, no favours – and, most assuredly, no giving way to the other guy. He was in the driving seat. He had 295 points to my 291, with Vermeulen on 282 – but, in reality, it was going to be a showdown between me and Laconi. No one else. And it would all take place on the Frenchman's home turf. Winner takes all ...

Eleven

WE ARE THE CHAMPIONS

I would have walked over anybody, done anything, and been as ruthless as any other guy set to post history and who was poised to wear a world championship crown. I felt it was MY title, my red-letter day: 3 October, 48 hours before my 24th birthday.

We headed for the climax of the season to Magny-
Cours, the odds, most people seemed to believe,
firmly stacked in Laconi's favour and against me. The
four-point advantage he had as championship leader, they
argued, would be hard for me to make up and he would
be all fire, fury and passion personified, taking the title on
his home ground for a French win. Everyone knew this
was going to be the dramatic and fitting end to what had
been a gripping season of toing and froing at the top. One
thing was certain, one of us was going to come away
heartbroken – and I vowed to myself it wasn't going to be
me. Not having got this far and having suffered and
sacrificed so much in the cause of championship glory.

I didn't reckon third-placed Chris Vermeulen, despite
the mathematical possibility, had any real chance of
robbing me of the crown. And despite Laconi's lead, I
knew deep down inside it was not all over and done with.
The French fans' belief that it was a foregone conclusion
was, if I had my way, going to be rammed back down
their throats. I think I scared myself with the strength of
my own resolve and the increasing intensity of my
determination not to come this far only to finish up
second. Formula One McLaren boss Ron Dennis refers to

second place as 'the first of the losers', scathingly dismissing runners-up, and that kind of summarised how I felt.

The previous year I'd had to come from nineteen points behind to pip Laconi for third place in the championship. And I still beat him. This year, the margin was a lot less to shut down. I felt, without wanting to sound cocky, that I had the upper hand mentally and, anyway, I was confident I was good and quick around the French track. How many more advantages could I take to the line?

The tensions of the last half of the season had really started to get to me. I recognised changes in my whole attitude. My mum and the rest of the family noticed it, too. I looked drawn and was very insular, fiercely determined, and focused as never before about my individual races. I could only think about my overall target, and just wanted to escape from everything else, preferring my own company. I reminded myself all the time that this was my chance to be a champion ... the WORLD champion – the best in the business. I dreaded the notion of coming second and having to go to those out-of-season promotional gigs and motorcycle shows and be introduced: 'And here's the WSB championship runner-up, James Toseland.' No, no, no.

I stayed on in Italy after the Imola round, not to avoid people, but because it was good to relax, and then flew straight to France for the race. It would have been too messy, and not at all sensible, to fly back home after Italy on Monday and then take off again for Magny-Cours on Wednesday. I was feeling refreshed, but totally charged for the task to come, when I arrived at that quiet little country village. The team completely took over the hotel where I was staying with my personal trainer Dave Marshall. Dave had been with me at the two previous races at Assen and Imola and was expert at preparing me physically – and he was a wonderful sounding board for me, too. He was older than me at 42, but he was wicked company and clever at getting me to talk about things other than motorbike racing: women, boozing, lads stuff.

It was all intended to keep my mind off the dangers and keep me from worrying too much about the race 24/7. His chats, late into the night when I couldn't sleep too well, kept me on track for the upcoming set-to, and helped me relax without taking the edge off my motivation.

I had got myself into a surreal state; I was so switched on I would have walked over anybody, done anything, and been as ruthless as any other guy set to post history and who was poised to wear a world championship crown. I felt it was MY title, my red-letter day: 3 October, 48 hours before my 24th birthday. All the pieces were in place: my first year in a factory team, my first real chance to leave my mark in motorcycle race folklore. Those long and lonely hours of painstaking and all-out sweated effort in the gym, setbacks that everybody kept reminding me would have made a less committed guy crumble, and the love and support of my mum, family, the team and all my friends had come down to this. I was racing not only for the title, but for my future.

My aim was to take control from the very first firing up of my motor, from Friday morning. There was no rocket science behind my thinking. My plan: go fast – then faster in the afternoon – grab Saturday by the scruff of the neck, morning and afternoon, and show ahead of race day that I was going to be the man to beat. In qualifying, a hot-paced rehearsal for the big show, I hit the front row of the grid, barely a thousandth of a second from being the pole-sitter, but still with my mark on the track truly registered. The look on my face, a mask of blank, unsmiling focus, was a dead giveaway – I meant business.

Over breakfast on race day, at about 7.30 a.m. in the team's hospitality area, I thought back, slightly smugly, about the frenzied action at Laguna Seca. Laconi and I had a real heart-in-mouth dice that had seen him childishly throwing his toys out of the pram when we got back to the motorhome we were sharing in the paddock. I fancied that I had him out-psyched from then on in.

In that race I had travelled backwards from first to fourth because of a tricky tyre problem that put the skids under my chances in race one. The situation sagged from bad to worse – and it was Laconi who kept me off the podium. I was really pissed off about the tyre issue and I made up my mind, come hell or high water, not to be shoved off the podium again. And my attitude triggered a bitter battle that carried through to the second race. Laconi came by me but went wide, so I dived under him. Then he passed me once more, but went wide again, so I got him back. His tyres, I could see, were better than mine so I realised that if he got ahead he would have pulled away with little I could do about it. So it became a case of 'Let Battle Commence'. I wired myself up for a confrontation. He came past again, I got the lead back straight away and he was on my outside, so I picked the bike up, with him stranded there, and headed for the gravel going as wide as I could and sort of shepherding him into the mucky stuff. I didn't have to do that, I still had the racing line, but I deliberately put myself in his way to have him off the track, not deep in the gravel, but just onto the dirt so I could keep him behind me. I thought it was a great race, very exciting and ballsy. However, the debacle had upset him and with typical Latin reactions he let his temperament take over. Back in the motorhome, when we were getting out of our leathers, he was angrily throwing his stuff around and banging about all over the place. The team manager, Davide Tardozzi, had to come in like a boxing referee – no biting, no gouging, no punches below the belt. Not that Régis would have squared up to me. He is emotional, but not a fighter.

My opinion of my tactics was that I didn't really do the dirty on him. I admit the manoeuvres I was pulling on him were tough, but they were designed to overcome my tyre disadvantage and I just kept getting in his way. I wanted so much to beat him in that second race, more or less at all costs. I reckoned I was ruthless – but not reckless. Even so, if TV had been showing our scrap for third place, instead of tracking the leaders who had cleared off, as often happens when two guys get caught up in a personal tussle and slow each other down, I might have been in trouble. Particularly if they had pictured some of the naughtier action. It certainly was not the brightest situation for two guys from the same team to be risking finishing in a gravel trap just to settle a personal squabble. But it had been that sort of weekend. The Laguna antics could not have done anything to damage a friendship. There was not one. We have never socialised beyond a bit of chitchat if we were attending a team meal. On the track, he is just another rider to be beaten. Tough.

What with our American stand-off, Régis and I have never been the best of buddies. A lot of his downfall is because of his emotional explosiveness – that's when he gets erratic and makes mistakes. Then, when it all goes awry for him, he weeps buckets, any ebullience drains out of him and he dejectedly moons around. If it has all gone good, he is a totally different fella. He's on springs, jumping about all over the place.

I can't be like that. And I suppose I have always been something of a puzzle to the Italian lads in the team. They can't figure me out because I never, if I can help it, let my emotions get the better of me: I am too self-contained, I don't often let the outside world in. That's why I don't get spectacularly and animatedly elated, leaping all over the place and screaming in triumph, when I have had a win. I may be bursting inside, but the reflection of my towering joy and personal satisfaction is usually nothing more than a smile. It's the same when I have been humbled in a race, either through my own doing or a fault of the bike's, or narrowly beaten. My response, however dejected I am, is not to try to take it out on anybody or point a finger in blame, but to swallow the upset and do my best to overcome it and not show my disappointment. That, I rule, is between me and myself, and for me to sort out in my own good time.

I didn't know how Laconi was handling the build-up to the last round, the decider; we both wanted to win, and I didn't care. There was no favouritism being shown in the garage, though both sets of mechanics, his and mine, were all right on the ball, and revelling on the fine edge of preparation the race was going to demand. A mechanical breakdown, for either one of us, through slack assembly or carelessness, would have been disastrous and unforgivable. We need not have worried. Everybody was on the case and the atmosphere in the garage had an underlying buzz that was catching. I wanted to do as well for all those guys with the spanners and stuff as I did for myself.

My pre-race regime, because I am such a creature of habit, is nearly always the same. I am happy if I have qualified well and a misery-guts if I haven't. I am usually concerned that there will be a need in the race, particularly from the start, to turn things around. If things haven't gone so well in qualifying I sit down with my engineer and we examine all the telemetry. It is a very painstaking effort to pinpoint the problem and find solutions. I am so familiar with the Ducati and its characteristics after five years that I can usually, roughly, outline what needs to be changed for the better. That's a useful scenario because it takes pressure off the chief engineer to find answers to the puzzles the bike can sometimes pose. In the old days racers used to have a catalogue of convenient and unchallengeable excuses why they had crashed or dropped a big clanger. Not now. The telemetry back in the garage has all the answers and, when you make up what you think is a clever excuse, the boffin monitoring all the graphs comes back five minutes later with a read-out in his hand saying, 'Oh, yeah – so when you fell off, it was nothing to do with you braking three metres later than you should have done, then?' Your smart-arsery counts for nothing then.

Then, if we are really struggling to find answers, and, say, Régis has gone better, we overlay his sheets and mine to see where he is making up the time and what I need to do to alter the situation. But, honestly, I prefer not to depend on the telemetry; I know what the bike feels like and how it should be reacting to my demands on it and I usually can tell, almost instinctively, what needs to be done to get it right. You can fine-tune the bike from the charts, but in the final analysis it all comes down to what a rider feels and how comfortable he is with its performance and balance. The engineer, as shrewd and as sharp as he may be, cannot feel what you feel when you're actually riding the bike. Luckily, with all my experience I am fairly good at getting my message across to the guys in the garage.

After we have gone through all that palaver, my routine follows its regular Saturday night pattern: I leave the garage and go to eat in hospitality – well, it is free and I am a Yorkshireman! I usually have a high-protein meal so that I am not too weighted down and bloated to get a good, unbroken night's sleep. I get all the carbohydrates and all the necessary energy sources through the day.

Before I take my rental car back to the hotel, as part of my contract I often have to mingle with some of the sponsor-related or Ducati VIP guests, signing autographs and posing for pictures, which can be fun and relaxing, but by now I am starting to switch my brain into gear for the race the day after and I guess I can look a bit distant and disinterested. I don't mean to and I suspect most people understand if I begin to yawn. The first thing I do when I get to my room is phone my mum, my grandma, my brother, my uncle, my former sponsor John Jones, who has become a firm friend, Roger Burnett, my manager, and all my pals, just to let them know how qualifying went, that I am OK and tomorrow (race day) is going to be fine and I am settled and confident about it.

Then it is wash-down time. I take a shower first and get all nice and clean from the sweaty mess from the day's action in a set of clingy leathers. If it is hot I have a stone-cold bath, sit in it for four or five minutes and let it take the lactic and all the other useless stuff out of my muscles. It's not as big a nightmare as you might think. Anyway, I soon get over the goose pimples.

Sunday – race day – and I get up at 7 a.m., early because we have a warm-up at 9.20 a.m., and have a light cereal breakfast. I never draw the curtains when I go to bed because I hate waking up in the dark – I just welcome the sun shining through the windows lighting up the room. It makes me feel good and alert right away; much better than if it is raining. I don't mind racing in the rain, but I always think when it is wet, it spoils the day for the spectators. It's just not nice.

I take a shower, then I go through a ritual of carefully strapping up the toes of my left foot with surgical tape and corn plasters as padding against the rubbing of the gear shift that can scrape all the skin off if you're not careful. On with the Ducati team livery over the boxer shorts I wear (because they are comfortable under leathers), and with a deep breath and a quick check-up in the mirror I say to myself: Come on, this is it, get yourself together. Thankfully, I am not hampered by superstition so I don't find myself, like so many other guys, doing things like not putting on my right boot before I have completed three handsprings in a southwesterly direction, or kissing myself on the back of my neck before I clamp my helmet on.

The traffic is normally thin going into the track at that time in the morning. I am usually safely parked and in hospitality, untroubled and unhassled, for 8 a.m. – that's if I haven't forgotten my paddock pass and left it in the hotel as I did at Assen, finding myself up against the tough and immovable gateman. Gatemen are not always car or bike fans, just somebody doing a job as a matter of work, as a change from guarding a brewery or a bank, so they don't always recognise the riders. Often, they do not know me from Adam. I could have argued that I am James Toseland, World Champion-in-Waiting, but anybody could claim that. And that was the problem I had with this massively burly Dutch guy when I forgot my car-park pass. He would not believe I was who I said I was and that I was racing that day. And not even the insistent support of a group of English fans who spotted me stranded in no-man's-land could persuade the jobsworth that I was a rider – even though I was kitted out from top to toe in team Ducati. It was ridiculous – there I was dressed in red from head to foot, trousers, shirt, shoes and cap. Who the hell would dress like that just to get in for free? Suddenly, against my usually calm nature, I lost my patience and flared. It didn't matter to me that he was about ten-feet tall and built like a windmill, I was about to go sailing in ... very ambitously, I may say. Luckily, for me I suppose, the team manager, Dave Tardozzi, finally answering my pleas by mobile phone, came to my rescue and probably saved me the embarrassment of being battered to death.

If I can, I like to watch the start of the race before ours, maybe the Superstocks, to see how quickly the race controller presses the button for the go-lights. I try and get some rough idea of the time-elapse he operates – anything, anything at all that might give me even a vital split-split-second advantage over the guys around me on the grid.

I take three sets of leathers with me to a race, but I prefer to wear ones that I have used before because by then they have moulded themselves to my contour. I'm not too keen on wearing new ones, they are always a bit tight and uncomfortable, but I will if I have damaged the suit in a crash or it has got wet in a rainy session and turned smelly. The makers measure you in the posture you adopt when you are riding a bike, so when you stand up normally everything tightens up and that can be a bit uncomfortable, especially around the nether regions. I have one set especially for the Italian races. They have Giacomino across the back instead of Toseland – it was the nickname given to me one day by a lovely girl, Sabrina, who works in the SBK offices. And it caught on. It means Baby James or Young James – Giacomo, like the legendary Italian champion Agostini's first name, stands for James and Bambino means Baby. Sabrina halved the two, then spliced them together for an affectionate nickname and I thought it would be a nice gesture to give something back to identify with all the Italian and Ducati fans who have been so kind and supportive.

By the time I have changed into my leathers in the motorhome, the boys in the garage have run up the bike, the tyre warmers are on and everything is all set to go. If we have had problems over the weekend we will probably try something in the morning run-out to solve it. I have a new engine in the spare stand-by bike and I do one lap on it to make sure it is hunky-dory in case we need to make a last-minute switch. Then I come straight back in to swap to my number-one bike, the one set up for the race proper, for the average twenty-minute, ten-lap session. Hopefully, by then, my times have been spot-on and steady so that I am well set up and in a positive mood for the rest of the day's work. You need good times in the morning to get yourself up to speed, and if you are comfortable, and the bike feels perky, then any other worries or doubts ebb away. What you are going to have to sit on and make work for two hectic forty-minute madcap runs, has to be as right as right can be. Not only that, it is crucial to your mental approach and your comfort zone, and as a boost to your confidence, that the equipment is as ready for the task ahead as is the rider.

The grid can be an absolute maelstrom of activity, packed with people, some who should be there, some who definitely should not: hangers-on, blaggers of VIP passes, show-offs and hordes of wanderers around who just seem to want to be part of the shows. Fans are a different matter, but these people are not even interested in the sport, just as long as they can get their faces on television or in the magazines and newspapers that follow motorbike racing. I prefer it when the five-minute klaxon goes and everybody is cleared off the grid and you can hear the murmur, the buzz, of the crowd in the grandstands as they settle in their seats.

On the start line all of us racers are trying to look cool, calm and unflustered before the nerve-jangling, throat-filling countdown. The mechanics unravel the tyre warmers, glance over their shoulders as a final check on the rubber, and their rider, and hurry away tugging tool trolleys and all the paraphernalia they need to keep their show on the road. I sit back in an eerie sort of solitude, stare down the now-quiet track that in just a few short minutes will be a bedlam of rushing, darting, diving, screaming machinery with riders, bursting with self-belief. Every single one of us is right on, and over, the edge, knowing that there is no way we will back off or yield one inch, however tight and fierce the racing gets.

Now, with time ticking away until we go, we have reached the point of no return. I just feel as if I am on the brink – striving for the ultimate, about to test my skill to the limit and wondering whether the bike can withstand what I have in mind for it. I reach a point where I have totally given myself to the race that is about to happen – I have let the will to win totally take over. That's when the last man to leave my side, Gabrielle, my chief mechanic – a tiny guy with the little-man's disease of being terrier-like and aggressive – usually grabs my gloved hand and growls in his odd Italian-English accent, 'Be angry, James, be ANGRY.' And I just give him a wink.

By then I can't wait to get going. There is an explosion waiting to happen deep down inside me and at the end of the warm-up lap I ram home to myself that I have got to fire myself off the line and be as aggressive and as forceful as I can.

On the starting line at Magny-Cours for this 2004 showdown, I noticed that, as usual, Regis had gone flat out from the last corner and slammed his brakes hard on. I don't know why he always does that, maybe to warm up his tyres or get a feel for the bike. But it does look erratic. Chris Walker, too, is doing his habitual trick of gawping around. Momentarily, and ludicrously, with the championship there for the taking and with my dreams of claiming it soaring sky-high, I am worrying if the television cameras picked up my swallowing a jelly baby just before I shut down my visor. My trainer, Dave Marshall, used to feed me Jaffa Cakes and jelly babies as energy supplements and he gave one to Julian Thomas, our press officer, who comes on the grid before the race, to pass on to me. He unwrapped this little green thing and I popped it in my mouth – then I thought: Bloody hell, if telly picked that up it will look really dodgy, as if I'm popping a pill or something.

Being the Frenchman in France and with such inescapable attention everywhere he went, Laconi was under enormous pressure. I knew it would be to my advantage, and qualifying fifth did not help his cause. He was, probably, from that moment on the back foot. We were pulled together in the garage before the race and ordered not to rough each other up and to keep it clean. No cutting each other up or barging. As if . . .

Nothing was going to stop me being champion – that was my goal and I was in the mood, with exactly the correct mindset, to achieve it. I had come too far to miss out. Not Laconi or any other rider was going to keep my hands off the World Superbike crown.

Then it was the set-off: I got away fast and made the holeshot, but Troy Corser snatched the lead until I reclaimed it at the hairpin. Haga squeezed by me and Laconi moved to fourth place, so he was still a threat. Haga and I, going hell for leather, came close to touching – but I eased away, only slightly, by 0.4 seconds. Haga regained the lead and set the fastest lap as Laconi and Vermeulen traded positions. I got to the front again, this time with Laconi passing Haga to nip into the second spot and start closing me down. The Japanese got Régis back and I led by 0.9 seconds. Poor old Chris Vermeulen stopped with engine problems after eleven laps – meaning he was out of the title chase. That left me and Laconi making it a two-horse face-off for the championship.

On lap fourteen he went wide in his dice with Haga's 999 – and that gave me a bit of a breather with a one-second lead. Troy Corser was next to suffer. He had to quit a lap later with mechanical problems. I headed for home with a 1.5-second advantage over my team-mate, but with Haga giving me a hard time and Laconi refusing to surrender. On lap 19 of 23 there was only half a second separating the 3 front-runners, but on lap 21, I got my head down and Haga and I squirted it for the flag and left Laconi somewhere in our wake, with me just beating Nori for the opener's points.

Going into the last lap was surreal. As I aimed for the finish, ten yards after the last corner, I stared hard at the man with the chequered flag to make sure I hadn't lost count of the laps and he was holding it to signal the end of the race. I just put my head in my hands in a mixture of disbelief and relief. It was like an action replay of the soaring feeling I'd had going for the title in the last lap of the 1995 Junior Road Racing Association championship at Mallory Park. That's how much motorcycle racing means to me – whatever title, schoolboy, junior, local, national, European or world, the sensation, the sense of satisfaction through personal endeavour, is the same. This realisation was no different from any other championship success: I am actually going to do this . . . I am going to be champion. There was, of course, a second leg to come, but I was filled with the certainty that I had done it. Even now, when I watch it on video, I could burst into tears with the perfection of it all.

There was a couple of hours, an agonisingly long wait, before the second session. I got out of my leathers and had a massage and a stretch in our motorhome, making sure I ate well enough to keep my energy levels sparking, with water to rehydrate and a cup of coffee to get some caffeine into my drained system. Because I was in France and was robbing a French guy of the title, there was not much back-slapping; everybody was rooting for Regis and I am sure that made me even more fired up to do the business.

However, my family were there to support me, and that was all that mattered. My brother, his partner Kirsty and my nephew Bailey were right there when I pulled up from the cooling-down lap after the opening race and he was in tears. I gave Simon a hug – but it did not register with me that the job might be finished – and I wasn't comfortable with him crying. I wanted to tell him to pull himself together and slap him around the face, but his joy, and his pride in his kid brother, was so overwhelming I didn't have the heart to be critical.

The second race, the clincher, was another humdinger, with Nori Haga and I again giving it some stick ahead of Régis. Troy Corser was quick off the mark – but I got him by the hairpin and went through, chased by Vermeulen on the Honda Fireblade. Laconi was still in the mix, up to fourth, but then he went wide and it became a thriller of a race between me, Haga and Vermeulen. It then went Nori's way and he stretched us out behind him. Steve Martin had to pull out from fifth spot with a mechanical problem and then Vermeulen's French jinx struck again on lap eighteen, so he had to retire. Corser had dropped away, and so had Chris Walker, who finished eighth in both races. I wasn't going to do anything stupid and as long as I kept Laconi behind me in third place, I was content to let Haga clear off for a win and leave me to grab the real glory, the World Superbike title. Laconi's threat faded as his heart went out of the challenge and, despite the scare of nearly getting knocked off by a back marker 2 laps from the end of the 63-mile race, I kept him well in the distance. I had a minor worry with the front tyre and was having to concentrate to keep the bike upright through the corners. And just to keep the wear and tear down on the gearbox I was short-shifting going along the back straight. On the last lap I was travelling so slow, drumming 'safety first . . . safety first' in a head that was buzzing with excitement, that I nearly stalled it at the hairpin.

I had a good long look over my shoulder and saw I was safely home, well clear of Laconi – and by then my eyes had filled up to the point where I could hardly see where I was going and I nearly crashed. I did burn-outs and wheelies and waved and thumbs-upped the crowd. When the chequered flag had fluttered in confirmation of my second place and signalled me as the youngest-ever winner of the WSB world championship, I burst into tears and cried streams all the way round the cooling-down lap. The outpour was simultaneous with the realisation that all my dreams had been laid out before my eyes. I had just about dried up by the time I rode into the throng in the winner's enclosure. Mum was there. Somehow she had climbed over the fence and fought her way through the mob crowding around my bike and was crying so much I started to fill up again. She was hugging me and shouting, 'You've done it!' That's all I recall her saying. I couldn't say anything in return, I couldn't respond, because I couldn't get my breath. Then she disappeared. I don't know where she went, whether she had been ordered to leave or had just gone and left me to it or what, but I just wanted to give her a big hug back. She was my number-one fan and had travelled the world to be at the tracks, even though she couldn't bring herself to watch me race. Usually, she only viewed the last lap, going for walkabouts or sitting in the hospitality or motorhome during the rest of the race. Magny-Cours was the first time she had watched it all.

I was wrecked, emotionally drained, and hardly able to comprehend the magnitude of my achievement. I had longed for this day – I had followed the World Superbike legend Carl Fogarty and my good friend Neil Hodgson as a British world champion. I slumped over the bike and then pulled myself together and stood triumphantly on the petrol tank like a stunt rider, helmet still on, and waved my arms in the air, forefingers forming a figure one, in what was both a self-salute and a tribute to everybody who had featured in my success. My chief mechanic shoved his head between my knees and hoisted me high in the air. And with that, the party had started . . . I looked at the masses of British people, with my tearful family and friends, cheering, yelling, waving and celebrating all around me, then noticed all the French fans filtering disappointedly out of the paddock. Laconi, to his credit, came across and offered his congratulations with a handshake. The feelings I had mounted in a crescendo of pride; so few sportsmen have the unique and unforgettable experience of being hailed as the best in the world, the champion. When you climb the podium, are hailed as the ultimate winner and hear your national anthem, there is no sensation quite like it. I knew in that instant what countless Olympians, World Cup winners, Grand Prix drivers and motorbike race title-holders have all felt and it gives me tingles up and down my spine even now. It was such a memorable and humbling moment when the strains of the anthem echoed over the masses that had turned respectfully silent as they thronged beneath the podium. I will carry the vision of the crowd – some still smiling, others even weeping – for ever more. I can't imagine that there is any other experience out there that can match that level of emotion – maybe having kids.

I scanned the crowd for familiar faces and there seemed to be hundreds of people, some just acquaintances and others foreign friends without a word of English beyond a friendly 'hi', who had travelled this long and very tough and challenging journey with me in some way or another with varying levels of closeness since I was first in a world-championship paddock in 1998. I hoped my waves and acknowledgments could be some small representation of the big thank-you I owed them for their unfailing support. They had all put such faith in my ability to get to the top. Sure, I'd had some really disappointing mid-season mishaps and the lowest of lows, bad results and crashes. A few doubters began to question my capabilities, and I needed real friends to lift me through those darker moments, and they did. I was so grateful for their continuing trust in me. And on the day, when the finale was in full flood, I had so much belief in myself, so much focus, I did not imagine, even for one second, that I could possibly make a mistake. If that sounds cocky, I apologise. But in all honestly I had to teach myself to have superior thoughts and be unfazed when things failed to go the right way; like yelling at myself to get a move on when I watched myself on television having a rotten race. That learning curve never seems to end.

Two of the first reactions to my championship came almost immediately from Carl Fogarty and Neil Hodgson, who was having an awful struggle in his switch to MotoGp but who still found time in the midst of his own lows to send me a message of congratulation. Neil was holidaying with his wife Kathryn in Langkawi, Malaysia, when he received confirmation of my success. And he sent back the message: 'I am chuffed to bits. What James did took balls because when it all hinges on the last race the pressure is immense. And then it is a case of who has the guts to go for it. And he certainly had – and did. He has been given nothing. He has had to fight for every scrap, every yard of the way and that is why I respect him so much. What with Foggy and me taking the world titles, and now James, the run of great British bikers has been kept going. I expected nothing less because he is one of the most dedicated riders I have ever met. He has worked hard to get where he is and he has done it with self-belief, nerve and a massive amount of riding ability and genuine talent.'

Then he offered a real heartfelt warning to me, based, I suppose, on his sad experience: 'I don't know what offers you might have for next year – but if one of them is for MotoGp don't take it for the sake of it and just be making up the numbers, because that's a waste of time. Only do it if you are assured of a decent ride.'

People have often joked that Carl Fogarty, four times the WSB champ, only ever felt it was worth opening his mouth about another rider if he could say something bad about them. OK, he is outspoken and not afraid to have an opinion that skirts political correctness, but he was fulsome in his praise for my performance. And he said: 'When it mattered James stood up to be counted. Laconi must be kicking himself for the mistakes he made. To win the world title in your team-mate's backyard is really something else. I said Toseland would be champion one day – and here he is. The way he has ridden in the last three rounds I can't imagine Ducati will not want to keep him.'

There was no on-the-spot indication from the manager, Davide Tardozzi, that they were about to extend my one-year contract – unlike Laconi's which, I understood, promised him another deal with the factory Ducati Corse if he won the WSB championship. Still, I thought, I would just have to wait and see.

There was a suspicion that Davide and Ducati would have preferred Laconi to have taken the title, but I did not detect or suspect any feedback of favouritism myself. I was happy with the way they had looked after my interests and I was sure they appreciated that I emerged victorious fair and square. Tardozzi's glum look of disappointment after the race, with his mouth turned down at the edges, was, he insisted, misinterpreted and he was really quite pleased. 'I am very happy for James,' he said. 'It is correct that he wins the title because he makes fewer mistakes. As for my look, that is just my face and the way it is. Being a team manager is like being the father to two children – and I do not want to be too happy for one and pissed off for the other.' My manager, Roger Burnett, a former British champion and Isle of Man Senior TT winner in 1986, and as much my mentor as he is my manager, now had a second world-title winner on his CV. He had looked after and shaped Neil Hodgson's career. He was, in fact, away in Qatar in the Middle East over my race weekend. He was my spy thousands of miles away from the track. He kept in touch by mobile and fed me information, particularly about Laconi and where on the circuit he was either strong or weak, after each qualifying session he watched on television, then he gave me a pep talk before the race and spoke to me again between the two legs. He told me afterwards that he knew the way I was riding that day that there was no way I was going to be beaten for the championship. He said, 'When you won race one, then I was one hundred and ten per cent certain. I could tell by your attitude and your body language that you were switched on for the confrontation. There are plenty of people who have been in a position to win championships – but there are not a lot of people with the mindset to do it and finish the job off. And that is what has impressed me most about you.'

It took an age for it to sink in that I was the world champion – and back in my hotel room, after some serious celebrating late into the night at the track, I woke up wondering if it had all been a dream ... and there, making it all positive, were the streams of sunlight guiding my red-rimmed eyes and pointing to reality. I had three glinting magnificent trophies, including one for the championship that weighed 20 kg. In a couple of hours, they were about to earn me a penalty of payment as excess baggage. Aren't airlines wonderful at bringing you right back down to earth?

Twelve

DON'T LOSE YOUR HEAD

I would have hated my win to have drained into anticlimax; it was the one priceless prize I had always cherished and I wanted to keep the satisfaction and thrill of it right at the top of my agenda. I did not let myself down.

When I arrived back in Sheffield the next day, a day before my 24th birthday, I just wanted to get back to a normal home life, and see all my old mates, as soon as I could. For my birthday celebration, we went down the road to my local pub, the Half Moon, for a steak dinner. My gran was there. I'd wanted to see her because she hadn't been able to make the trip to France to see my championship decider – and it was a very emotional experience for both of us with lots of proud smiles and tears, too, of joy and relief. I suppose after all the hard chasing and the crashes, she was glad I was still in one piece. I don't think Gran would have worried whether or not I'd won the title – but, of course, was thrilled about it – just as long as I was OK, safe and happy with whatever I had chosen to do with my life.

I was so overwhelmed by my achievement and the shock of it all, looking every day at the two trophies on my sideboard and making sure they were still there and not a figment of my imagination. I gave myself special time for reflection in long moments of solitude at home. I played the piano late into the night and kept myself to myself, with only rare trips out, mainly to my mum's for something sensible and nicely cooked to eat instead of my usual takeaways.

I was quite content with my own company for a while. It was pleasant, relaxing and refreshing after the hectic roller-coaster ride my life had become leading up to that last big championship gamble, that last throw of the dice. However, I soon felt a desperate need to indulge in a bit of wild behaviour (and there are always a good few long-term pals around to help me out). I opted to do just that . . . in Las Vegas. It was a wicked trip. Just as wild as you would imagine in the world's maddest, glitziest, most extravagant 24-hour merry-go-round place on the planet.

I would have hated my win to have drained into anticlimax; it was the one priceless prize I had always cherished and I wanted to keep the satisfaction and thrill of it right at the top of my agenda. I did not let myself down.

I guess I have Neil Hodgson to thank for that with his unwillingness, if I can call it that, to whoop it up when he clinched the World Superbike title at Assen in 2003. He said there was no party afterwards and it might have been that his world-championship victory had, in his thoughts, been overshadowed by the birth of his first child, his five-day-old daughter, Holly. In its own way that had taken the edge off being champion, as it was more satisfying to him that he had become a father. That was proudly proclaimed when he peeled his leathers to his waist after his clincher in Assen and on a T-shirt under his kit was printed: 'Who's The Daddy?' The way he was talking afterwards was as if being the champion wasn't all it was cracked up to be and he wasn't too bothered and I thought, hang on a minute, he's the world champion and he is showing no excitement at all, he's not thinking about it – and that worried me. And that's why I felt: right, sod this, I'm going to Las Vegas.

It started that just my pal Matthew and I were going. I rang him up and asked, 'Do you fancy going to Las Vegas?' He said, 'I can't get time off work. Anyway, I'm saving up for a house.'

Blah, blah, blah.

So I said, 'It won't cost you. It's on me.'

He asked for time to think about my offer and was back on the phone inside thirty seconds saying, 'For free? I'm on.' Then, at a party at my house, the other lads, all drunk on my booze, said they wanted to come, too. My brother's girlfriend revealed that he was miffed and sulky because I hadn't invited him along and I explained I hadn't asked him because he had two kids and I didn't want to put him in an embarrassing situation.

She said she didn't mind – and the DJ at my party announced to massive cheers that Simon was yet another candidate for the nine-day booze-fest in Nevada. I flew a gang of about seven of us there, but they found their own spending money. I acted like any 24-year-old let loose with his brother and his mates: swilling beer until it came out of my eyes, gobbling pizzas at 3 a.m., clubbing, dancing and casino-ing up and down the Strip and staying up until first light. It was absolutely fantastic and just the fun I cried out for after so much unshakeable, and necessary, focus on becoming a world champion.

After all the attention at racetracks all over the world, it was a pleasant change to move around unrecognised as just one of the lads. I did have one brief interlude during the trip, a break from my anonymity, in a jam-packed piano bar. They held little auctions to have a tune played – and if you didn't like the song that had been suggested and bid more you could get it changed to your choice. One of our lads bid fifty dollars on the proviso, he insisted, that his mate James could play the piano. They said that for fifty dollars, buddy, he can play what he likes. And then, my pal told them I was the World Superbike champion – and it was announced over the microphone, much to my embarrassment. I played 'Walking in Memphis' and then a bit of rock'n'roll and, I have to say, it went down well and I got a great big cheer. But then, playing keyboards and singing with my own band Crash at gigs all over Britain I wasn't the least bit shy. I'm happy to play for my hundred pounds a gig – we do about fifteen a year – with lads who have become good friends: Warren, backing vocals and acoustic guitar; Paul, who won the TV show *Stars in their Eyes* as Billy Joel; lead singer Gav on drums; and me on keyboard and doing some singing and jigging about in what I imagine is a sexy turn-on for the girls. We were originally called Shazoom and wore biking gear, but we feared the name made us sound too camp so we renamed ourselves the much more macho Crash.

It's strange: when I look at myself, I seem to have two identities. I am one sort of guy when I am around bikes, introspective and focused, and then when I am in the company and atmosphere of the band I am much more lively and animated. I have a stage personality – and I hope that doesn't sound like I put on a false face just for the show. It's all just a natural progression for me to switch from the extremely serious guy I am when I am racing, in that high-pressure environment as a rider and a centre of attention, to the more happy-go-lucky and outgoing character I am in my alter-ego guise as a musician. It's nothing to do with the money: we play it for real and, I reckon, we are pretty good. Not recording stars – but who knows what might happen in the future? In the meantime we have played in front of some fairly big audiences, two to three thousand sometimes, and I really enjoy it. I even got to play with Jools Holland when he asked me along to a big show in July 2005 at Newmarket. There was an audience of 25,000 and it was magic.

Of course, Mum was treated to a holiday, too. Just as a little thanks, I decided to take her on a well-deserved break in the Cayman Islands. I pulled her leg, saying that we were going to Benidorm – and I got my manager Roger to rig up some dummy flight details for Alicante on the Costa Blanca, the airport that serves Benidorm. Mum was excited about the trip and went to the bank to buy 400 euros.

We got to Terminal 4 at Heathrow, the inter-continental long-haul starting-point, but because she does not fly so often she had no idea it was not the location to check in for Spain. And I just kept her occupied and talking in case she caught sight of the destination screens. The biggest threat to her finding out was when an airline supervisor sorting out passengers into the right lines for their destination asked me where we were going. I put my bag down and told mum to do the same and whispered to the British Airways guy out of her hearing as she bent down, 'The Caymans.'

Somehow, without her suspecting, we made it onto the big jet, into club class, with her still thinking we were off to Alicante and not twigging that jets this size don't go there. I had piles of brochures about Benidorm for her to read and then I started taking the mickey, putting my in-flight socks on, getting my toothbrush out and shoving earplugs in and she said, 'What do you think you are playing at? It's only a two-and-a-half-hour flight.'

I suspected that three hours into the flight she would get curious about how long it was taking, but I had planned my excuses and I was going to say the plane had only small engines and that is why it was really slow. The captain came on the intercom and apologised for our delayed departure, but explained that we would shortly be taking off for Nassau – you flew on from there to the Caymans. Mum panicked, 'We must be on the wrong plane. He said we were going to Nassau.'

I said, 'No, not all. What's happening is, there must be something wrong with the plane and he's just rung NASA the space agency to make sure everything is OK before we set off.'

She three-quarters bought my very feeble explanation – but just to make sure she belled the stewardess and asked her if we were on the right flight for Alicante. I thought the poor girl was going to have a panic attack thinking she had passengers loaded on to the wrong plane so I had to give way and admit to all that it was a surprise.

We stayed nine days. Needless to say, Mum was thrilled. She sunbathed and I trained like mad and in the

searing heat of the West Indies with my *Rocky* CD on tap.
I ran like a man possessed up and down the beach every
day. It was her birthday while we were there, but she
found it difficult to celebrate it because I was so focused
on the championship. I was in a frenzy, getting myself at
an absolute peak of fitness and she was worried that I
wasn't enjoying myself as much as I should have been on
holiday. But it was great that we could spend quality time
together – that did me good – and it gave me ample
opportunity to reassure her about my hopes and dreams
and how I could handle the build-up of pressure.

Racing has given me so much and has been so much in
my thoughts, that it can be difficult to find time to spend
with loved ones. I give as much as I can to be with them,
but there is not much room for anything else. A permanent relationship with a girl is not so appealing and could
in no way compare to the utter satisfaction and delight I
have experienced in my job. Because I am so constantly
busy I do not have that much time to spare on any sort of
an emotional or loving tie-up. Sure, when you are lonely,
you want companionship and some girl to love and are
always on the lookout for someone to give yourself to. But
I don't get time to be lonely. Anyway, the thrills, the high
peaks of emotion and all the shades of excitement that
racing gives me could never be matched by sex. No matter
who with. I hope that doesn't sound sad. But it is a
brutally honest admission.

I would hate to have any girl believe she was the be-all
and end-all of my life. In the future, yes, when my bike
racing is over and done with and danger no longer exists,
when temptations vanish with faded fame, and I have
more time to devote to another human's concerns other
than my own.

I have always felt that too much star treatment is no
good – not very healthy, not too good for your balance
and your priorities – and I have always tried my best not
to be affected by the adulation that seems to go hand in
hand with any level of celebrity. Being the world cham-

pion is one thing, a truly amazing achievement, but underneath the crown I am still, and always will be, James Toseland, a Sheffield lad without pretentions. You can, if you are not careful, get hooked on fame and finish up a very lonely, ignored and disliked person. I like that saying, I don't know by whom, that goes something like: 'Better hellos than goodbyes', meaning it is awful when people are happier to see the back of you than greet you.

There was a revealing article in the *Daily Telegraph*, written by Brendan Gallagher, that went some way to explaining the sort of demands I make on myself in pursuit of what I perceive to be perfection, or as near to it as I can get.

He followed me to Butlins for a show the band performed at a *Motorcycle News* weekend for petrol-heads – and about 3,000 turned up to the Red Room that was meant to hold about 2,000. They were overflowing the place in a massive crush when at about 9.30 p.m. we came on stage. Gallagher wrote:

If a boy-band manager signed him today, Toseland would make his first million by the end of the week. No rock star in Britain would get a more rapturous reception this year.

Watching Toseland prepare during the sound check is an education. Crash are a full-time professional band who take pride in their work and even for such an audience-friendly gig they spent well over 90 minutes setting up. Toseland is totally in synch with that attitude. At one stage he took a full 15 minutes setting the position of his mike absolutely right, changing the stand height 27 times on my count. Attention to detail is everything, just as it is when preparing the bike to race around a track at nearly 200 mph.

'It just wasn't comfortable,' concedes Toseland. 'I am never happy until absolutely everything is 100 per cent. I expect I drive some people to distraction, but

I have a real strong perfectionist streak running through me.'

Shades of Jonny Wilkinson, Toseland has that stillness and presence you associate with most top sports names. On stage, and on the racetrack, he takes care of all the basics and the routine technical stuff and makes sure the number is nailed or the race won before indulging in any flash showboating.

Suzi Perry, the lovely Suzi, frontline voice of BBC TV's motorcycle race shows – and who really does know her racing stuff – had some nice things to say about me in the article. And, at the risk of blushing, I will quote her: 'He is one of the most charismatic sportsmen I have met. I was down in La Manga for the filming of *Superstars* and it wouldn't be unfair to say that on the first day none of his fellow competitors, or any of the spectators, had heard of him. By day two he was the ringleader and the focus of all the attention. Not that he deliberately sets out to achieve any of that, it just happens. I see it everywhere on the Superbike circuit. He is star material pure and simple, but there has also been years of hard work and heartache behind his overnight success. James is a very mature and tough lad – in the nicest sense – underneath it all.'

Steady on, Suzi . . .

I reckon there are natural links between racing and rock 'n' roll – being a biker and a keyboard player in a band is not such a strange contrast. Biking *is* rock 'n' roll and, in many ways, they are inseparable. One follows the other. I frequently take a bend or get my head on the tank on a long straight with a particular song or piece of rock music going through my mind. On stage I am focused and exact, but my timing has to be dead right, the same as when I'm on a bike racing. In both cases I strive to flow and be relaxed and easy and comfortable in what I am doing and what I am trying to achieve. That sort of process is recognisable to any top world-class rider about racing – or any musician, too, if he wants to get it right and play

214

memorable stuff. And, just like getting as much time in as you can on a bike, it is crucial to put all the hours you can spare into music and mastering your own particular choice of instrument until you reach the point, where all the moves are natural and second nature. Whenever I book into hotels, the first thing I do is check if they have a piano lounge. If the manager or the customers enjoying a few drinks don't mind, after practice or qualifying, I like to get a singsong going with a few Elton John or Billy Joel numbers. It is the perfect way for me to relax and dump the stresses that can build up at the track. For 2005 those pressures would be all about wondering and worrying whether I was going to get another contract out of Ducati, so that I could defend my championship, or move over to MotoGp. It was going to be a waiting game and I would have to make the most mature decisions of my life.

I did not have to hang on too long before the offers began to stream in. My manager, Roger Burnett, had been busy behind the scenes with his usual level of advanced wisdom. Based on the disastrous season of his other client, my old team-mate and pal Neil Hodgson, who had suffered in a switch to MotoGp, he reckoned, quite rightly, that unless I got a super offer from a frontline team – proven winners – I would be better off staying put in WSB. I fancied the idea of defending my title with Ducati and, anyway, the MotoGp deals on the table were not nearly as promising as we would have hoped for. Neither were the offers to quit Ducati and ride elsewhere, even though the money would have been better. Lots of teams, other major manufacturers, were heading back into WSB either with fully backed works or satellite outfits and, naturally, they would all have preferred to be displaying my Number One plate on their bikes.

To be honest, I rated myself a Ducati man through and through. I had grown up with the team, I knew the people and the way they worked, their moods and foibles, and I was content with my status and the way I was treated. And, as an added bonus for an always-hungry lad like me,

I enjoyed the food in hospitality. So I was happy to re-sign, though I did not put pen to paper until the season had got under way. That was the level of mutual trust that I and Ducati shared.

It sounds big-headed, but at this time, my confidence in my ability coincided with my championship trophy that I was the best – certainly for that year. Nobody had gifted me any favours, nobody had lay down, surrendered and said over to you mate, the title is yours. And I find it impossible to describe the satisfaction, without sounding smug, that I get all the time from knowing that if it never happened again I proved, at least to myself, that I did have the talent and drive to come out tops in an extremely tough, demanding and dangerous championship.

Just in case I did let it slip my mind that I was the reigning world champion, I always had my then five-year-old nephew, Bailey, who had been in France for the clincher, to gaze up at me from under his oversized Ducati cap when we were sitting at home and say with pride, 'You are the best . . . better than anybody in the WHOLE world.'

Outside that familiar environment of home and family I can, and still do, get a little embarrassed when I am recognised and I can't get my head around other celebrities' big I-AM attitudes and desperation to feed on whatever fame they have or imagine they have.

I was at a pal's stag party, very drunk, when a bloke, equally plastered, wandered up to me saying, 'Are you James Toseland, the motorbike racer?'

'No, pal, no way,' I answered, 'I'm Dave, a plumber.'

I am desperately anxious not to be seen to be taking advantage of whatever bit of fame I have. It's the same when I am out with my mates, I just want to be one of the lads, a regular guy enjoying a pint and a giggle, and not the hero they sometimes want to go on about to the point where, even though they are being nice, I am still uncomfortable listening to them. The closer the person to me, and Mum is nearest of all, if they start to discuss with friends in front of me what I have achieved I try to put a stop to it right away. I don't know whether that is a silly reaction or what. Truth to tell, I would rather just get on with the sort of conversation normal family and friends have – talking about fun times, holidays, the weather, politics, sport, girls, or merely gossiping in general.

Thirteen

THE SHOW MUST GO ON

I was irritated by some sections of the media, and some so-called race insiders who were writing me off, as if I was a one-season wonder. Rather than punish myself or waste time worrying about remarks like that, I would much rather get on with it.

The way the season in defence of my title went, or at least began, I was close to changing my priorities. In a word it was crap. You know the old saying about what you are left with after the Lord Mayor's show? I had to seriously remind myself of the passion I have for racing and not let the temptation to give up take over.

I'd had a nasty crash testing in Qatar, the biggest high-side of my career, the week before the start of the season. To add to that, come the start of the race, I was battered and bruised because of a bit of dune-buggy safari-ing, which I thought would be some way of finding escape and relaxation. Being driven by a madman who seemed barely in control as we leaped with alarming, bone-shaking zeal from one massive sandy hump to another, mostly on two wheels, head, back or side first, was not what I had in mind.

I was all fired up for Qatar, but I qualified a disappointing thirteenth, and in the races scored two sixths that were one hell of a battle in a rare downpour of rain. I just could not get the bike to hook up. We had new settings – it was set-up for five gears all weekend but we changed it to six for the race to try to get the front tyre to last the trip. By the end of race two, in which there were crashes all over the place, I was the fastest man on track, but by then it was far too late for me to improve my position. I had some real edgy hold-your-breath moments nosing in under people for passes that were, shall we say, a little bit squeezy. I realised that the advantage we had enjoyed the season before, with one of the fastest bikes on show, was all wiped out: the 999 Ducati was as good as any other bike, but it most certainly was not any better. The series was packed with good bikes and riders to greater depth but, I emphasised to myself, they were not unbeatable. Even so, I realised I was going to have to work hard and hope that the bike and the team could match my ambitions for them both.

Troy Corser, aged 33, got himself on track for the title with a win – his first in WSB for 4 years – in race one ahead of Yukio Kagayama's Suzuki with my team-mate Régis Laconi third. Race two saw Yuki win with Laconi second and Corser third. I had slipped to fifth in the championship.

Being a lousy, lowly thirteenth in the next testing at Valencia and crashes, including two horrendous high-sides at the Spanish track, set me back. I was left fuming that if ever I finished that far down the place and time sheets again I would pack it all up and go back to the piano as a career. I told myself I might be thirteenth fastest man in Valencia, but in WSB I certainly was not. However, I am not a quitter and I have come back from a lot worse. Troy Corser had registered his championship intentions and aspirations, and showed how quick and reliable his Suzuki was. Not only that, the Yamahas and Hondas were demonstrating some mighty and trouble-free pace.

At Phillip Island in the next round, Corser clinched a great double – and I had an absolute disaster which left me raging, particularly at Australian Karl Muggeridge's recklessness. He had carelessly ram-raided my friend Chris Walker the race before in Qatar, and apologised. But then he did the same thing to me Down Under. On lap five in race two, I was ahead of him and I heard him lock up his front tyre – then he hit me side on and put me out of the race. I was so mad I branded him 'shit'. I said at the time: 'He is erratic when he is riding in the pack – he leaves his braking too late and you can see him panicking. His race craft is shit. He did the same to Chris Walker in Qatar.'

He pleaded innocence and argued that I had been having some tough moves put on me and I was giving them back twice as hard.

'We were side by side,' he tried to explain, 'on the brakes, and James just let it run on a little and then truly shut the door on me. He left me no room. I tried my best to avoid him but I had nowhere to go, there was no more track left.'

It was just part of a stinker of a weekend. I had struggled with the rear tyre – it was spinning like crazy after only a couple of laps and I was lapping two seconds slower than I had done in qualifying. It was just a ridiculous mess of a race for me because the wrong rubber had been fitted and I fumed. I reckoned, with some justification, that it was not acceptable. Now I had to face a wearying 26-hour flight home with plenty to occupy my thoughts, and concerns, en route.

The Valencia jinx that seemed now to be hanging over me took another bite out of my title chances and, as early in the season as the race was (only round three), I could see my aims of a successful defence were going to be hard-earned. I scored just eight measly points – an eighth and a nineteenth. I got away 23rd in race 1 after a really rotten and disappointing qualifying caused by a puncture, probably the worst any reigning champion had ever cut. I even failed to make the line for the Superpole showdown and, through dint of sheer effort and a lot of chance-taking, managed a half-decent recovery to salvage a handful of points for eighth. In race two I got caught up in a crash caused by Garry McCoy (another Aussie) and then suffered a problem with the front wheel. It kept locking up and I had to pull in for repairs. I got back into the race, but to my intense disappointment and anger finished nineteenth, miles behind Corser who twice rode home ahead of Chris Vermeulen to complete a double on what he claimed was the best bike he had ever ridden. He boasted he wasn't even trying and had rolled off the power ten laps from the finish.

My title tally was a meagre thirty points and I was in tenth place with all these riders ahead of me: Corser and Kagayama on their brand new, all-conquering 205 bhp Suzuki GSX-R1000s, Vermeulen, Laconi, Norick Abe, Max Neukirchner, the German, Haga, Andrew Pitt and Chris Walker – all guys I had beaten before. I could see my crown was in danger of slipping even though I always class myself as a fighter, somebody able to pull a little extra out of the bag when it most matters. I knew that this could be a case of damage limitation from hereon in. We were taking too many gambles on things we shouldn't, but I didn't want to blame anybody but myself.

I could not, for the sake of team harmony, say much about the issues behind the scenes that were hampering my efforts – but, clearly, things were not going exactly to plan. I felt I was riding OK, going very well in fact, but a mix of mechanical puzzles, some wrong decisions, and trying to cope with tyre setbacks, all conspired to put the skids – literally – under my hopes of retaining the title.

A newspaper, citing a source close to Ducati, pinpointed what they believed was part of the problems I had to endure and overcome: the introduction of traction control. They revealed that the root of my problems this season could be the result of an electronic bug in the Ducati's traction control system that caused me to highside at 140 mph in Qatar. They said it appeared that the traction control was switched on, but failed at one of the fastest corners, causing a massive crash that destroyed my confidence in the system – and the bike.

The report added that a Ducati insider had said: 'The crash was not his fault. The system failed and James was thrown off the bike. He hasn't trusted it enough to switch it back on, but he realised at Valencia there was no option after failing to get into Superpole because of wheel spin.'

Ducati admitted it had fitted MotoGp-style electric traction control to my 999 as a device to regulate the formidable wheel spin that I was having to try to overcome and yet still try and be competitive and run with the leaders.

It didn't need the brain of Einstein to figure out that I was heading for a real trial of a season. Now that the 1996 champion Corser, 33-years-old, but a clever old fox of a rider who had lost none of his speed or ambition, had got his act together aboard a blisteringly quick Suzuki, my problems hanging onto that cherished Number One plate were increased double-fold. But I am no pushover and I am always up for the battle – just like my inspirational Rocky movies, where he takes on the bigger opponent, looking like the underdog and taking a few beatings, and then coming good off the back of his own determination. I was prepared to dig deep, and take chances, to find the necessary element to get me back in the fray as a front liner. I was irritated by some sections of the media, and some so-called race insiders, who were writing me off, as if I was a one-season wonder. Some cynics sniped that I was only a good national rider and I was lucky that I could play the piano. Rather than punish myself or waste time worrying about remarks like that, I would much rather get on with it.

The fight back started at Monza where I clawed my way back from six seconds down to earn a third place. With Silverstone coming up, allied to massive expectation from the British fans, I was going to be a force to be reckoned with and give it my absolute all. We tested for three days at Mugello, near Florence in Italy, right after Monza and I blitzed the time sheets and was 1.4 seconds faster than I had been the year before.

The way this private test worked out and the way the bike was behaving gave me a mega-boost for Silverstone.

It filled me with confidence. Up until then, the Ducati had not felt like a winner. We needed to work on the gearbox ratios because the Pirelli tyres would only operate satisfactorily within a certain rev range and we had not always had the best or most suitable and efficient gearing to maximise on its power. Now we had got it running just about as we wanted I felt good; I could see a breakthrough ending my misery and, hopefully, ramming some wicked words back down some bile-filled throats.

The year before Silverstone had been a shocker for me. Painful, too. I'd had just one podium in three years at the old wartime airfield track near Northampton and was looking to make amends in 2004. But a front-end crash nearly flat-out at Abbey in the opening race, well on the 150 mph mark, left me knocked about for the second leg and I wrote the weekend off as one of the most forgettable of my career.

I broadcast it far and wide to the doubters that there was nothing wrong with me, and nothing really amiss with the bike, but a run of bad luck had compromised my situation. I had nothing to lose and my feeling was that it was a case of no holds barred in front of what I knew would be a partisan crowd. I really hoped that it would be a big turnaround for me and the team.

My pal, Neil Hodgson, who knew a thing or two about comebacks and the need for fighting spirit, was a fine and firm supporter and, from America, where he was riding after his own disastrous year in MotoGp, said very kindly: 'One of James's biggest strengths is his mental ability – he has the character to pull positives from almost any situation. Whatever has happened, he will come out fighting. There were times in 2004 when it looked like it would all be over for him – but he ended up winning the championship. In a ding-dong battle I'd put my money on him every week.'

I was certainly in the right mood when I pitched up at Silverstone with 80,000 people packed in and all hoping for a classic. I wanted desperately to show them I was worthy of the Number One plate and I reckon I did – a third place in the first race set me up nicely to go two better in the second leg for my first win in Britain for seven years and my first triumph on home soil in the WSB championship. Among other changes, Ducati had abandoned the starter motors and some internal gears so they could redistribute the five kilos weight they saved: the crankshaft assembly, too, was altered so that the V-twin could rev more sharply and accelerate faster out of the corners to match the four cylinder bikes. I found the weight-saving beneficial and, at that stage, anything that helped give me some added performance was well worthwhile.

The first race fell to Laconi, who rode tremendously, with Corser second and me third. In the second leg, Haga, as he had done in race one, blasted out of the blocks ahead of Corser and Kagayama, with me watching the action from behind, but staying in touch. Laconi crashed at Woodcote Corner on lap two when the back-end broke away and tipped him off. By lap eight, Haga had outbraked Corser for the lead only for the Aussie to snatch it back straightaway as they exited Woodcote and hurtled down the long straight. I got Haga at Abbey with twelve laps remaining and then breezed by Corser a lap later, again at Abbey. Once I'd got ahead there was no way I was going to relinquish the advantage even though, with two laps to the flag, Troy had closed right up, but I wouldn't let him get close enough to make a passing move on me. And I romped home with the fans going mad – and me hardly able to keep back the tears. I was pleased for all the lads in the garage that Ducati had scored a double with me and Régis both beating Corser, the rider who was the pick of the championship on a Suzuki that had been shaping as truly awesome. From the standpoint of personal satisfaction, never mind for a moment the value of the points I had picked up, my Silverstone show gave me just the boost I needed to sustain my intention not to surrender the title without the sort of fight the other guys, my rivals, would all remember even if they beat me to the final high spots.

After the podium bubbly had been sprayed on my revitalised hope and I had waded through the acres of smiles, I said: 'The way I see it is that I've nothing to lose and everything to regain. I was fifth in the championship coming into the race – but fifth has no worth to me, it might as well be tenth. I tell myself I AM the world champion and I do not want to end up any lower than I did last year. Sure, Corser is a great rider on a very good bike and he will be an extremely difficult man to catch ... and pass ... in the chase for the title. But if Regis and I can keep the pressure on him, can keep pushing hard, like we both have done here at Silverstone you never know what might happen.'

Corser had run up 222 points, Kagayama was on 144, Vermeulen 141, Laconi, 112, with me on 98, 14 ahead of Chris Walker in sixth place. Corser said that in the race he welcomed the dice he'd had with me and Haga because we were not championship contenders and he said: 'At one point I got alongside James and could easily have let the brakes off and gone through, but he was coming across me and I didn't want us to touch. He was pushing harder than me but I am going for the championship – he was trying for his first win.'

My own joy was unbridled. 'Awesome,' was my excited response when I was asked how it felt to be a winner at Silverstone. And I added: 'People have been having a dig at me and asking questions about my ability. I feel, with this result and the one at Monza, I have answered them. It really does feel amazing – I have waited four years for this and it has been worth every minute. Last year, my aim was to win the world championship – and I did. This year my dream was to take a victory in the UK. And I have. My next target is to do the double at Brands Hatch.'

That, alas, was not to be. We had a brilliant two-day test session in Brno, in the Czech Republic, where, despite two crashes, I topped the time sheets ahead of Laconi,

Walker, Andrew Pitt and Haga. And at Misano, buoyed up by the Brno speeds and with a new 'idle speed control' system fitted, improved traction control and a hefty, extra-wide 200 mm rear tyre as against the regular 190 mm-width, I was in the right frame of mind to do a good job on Ducati's home ground on a boiler of an Adriatic day in front of a 60,000 crowd. But then Misano, just down the road from our Bologna HQ, has never really been too rewarding for me – and nothing changed in that regard. I managed two fourth places when I felt I should have done a deal better. To make it worse for me – better for Ducati – Laconi got two wins as I struggled to overcome front-end slides.

Our Ducati technical director Ernesto Marinelli revealed that the team had built two new electronic systems taken from the MotoGp bikes. And he explained: 'The first gives us the ability to control the idle speed for the corners and the second one is our own system which makes opening the throttle easier without spinning the wheel. Now our two riders can get on the gas on more lean. At Qatar, James had a major crash and lost confidence and it took time for him to get it back. Régis also had big crashes and people thought we were lost, but this is not true. Now we are getting the best out of our bike.'

In round seven, back in Brno, we had insurmountable problems with the tyres. Mind you, it seemed to be the same for the other teams, too, when Pirelli failed to get the required and necessary consistency into their supply. I was second in race one, after a fight from tenth place, and eighth in the second session, a race I felt I could have won if it hadn't been stopped because of an oil spill, then restarted. The team fitted new tyres during the break, but after three laps on the resumption they went haywire and I spent the whole time picking the bike up off the tarmac with my knee. It was there, I suppose, I first felt that my title was a gonner. Corser, with yet another win, was looking like the new champion and I wasn't too pleased.

It pissed me off big style and I made my feelings known to the press.

When I got to Brands Hatch, all nerves and determination, only to drop out of the first race with a crankshaft failure and then slump down among the also-rans in the second as Corser and Haga scrapped it out in two nail-biters, I suspected my title defence had failed. With 80,000 spectators out of their seats on the second race with excitement, the fans were maybe wondering what had gone wrong with me, let alone the bike. I was devastated.

With things going so badly wrong when I was riding as well, if not better, than ever before, I concluded I had to find the motivation to pick myself up and get on with life. I have had to contend with a lot of adversity, even from being a young boy, so there was no doubt in my mind that I already had that ability and I would continue to use it well.

Fourteen

I WANT TO BREAK FREE

I had registered my return to the top end of WSB with an impressive haul at Qatar, and a picture of my dogged determination and willingness to take chances was now firmly logged in the minds of my critics and the riders I was going to be up against for the rest of the season.

It was amazing how dramatically the atmosphere and situation changed in the Ducati camp. The highs of 2004 – the euphoria of the title triumph and the great, well-earned and sometimes hard-earned, victories – gave way in 2005 to a new succession of lows. I became aware that there were many people, even on home ground, who believed and wrote and said that I was a one-season wonder. That hurt. But it made me all the more determined to prove them wrong.

My own feelings of satisfaction and success carried me through the winter on the biggest high I could possibly have had, but I never once felt that it was my right as champion to be given any special treatment. I've always believed that I need to work hard and not sit back and expect people to give me anything for free.

Little did I realise that I was heading for a major setback in the shape of the scariest and fastest crash I'd ever had. At 152 mph on the fastest corner of the new Qatar track, the back wheel came round and snapped back, throwing me right over the high-side. I escaped – God knows how – with no broken bones, but I did suffer extensive and painful bruising, all over my body. I had blacked out when I went over the top, so when I somersaulted back to earth I was unconscious and as relaxed and loose as a rag doll. That stopped me tensing up in anticipation of being hurt and helped me escape serious injury. This happened just a week before the season began. I was lucky it wasn't a lot worse, but I was so disappointed because I had clocked some great times and had outpaced Laconi. The crash seemed to set the mark for what faded into a miserably disappointing and frustrating season, with a terrible Brands Hatch made all the worse by the expectations of about 100,000 British fans.

The 2005 season is thankfully history, but it was probably the saddest episode of my racing career. Behind the scenes, so many things seemed to be going wrong, technically and otherwise, and I felt as if I was battling against my own team. Every time I went into the garage I wanted to prove a point to the manager, the mechanics and the engineers. There wasn't actually a rift, but, ridiculous as it may sound, I almost felt as if I'd done wrong in winning the championship! It was certainly the first time I can remember when a winning team didn't celebrate on the day with a T-shirt proclaiming their victory.

Ducati had planned to send Laconi on a promotional trip to America for their last Superbike race of the season and, of course, it would have been great for them if he went as champion. It was already organised by the time I clinched the title at Magny-Cours, against all odds, so Laconi still made the trip. When I look back now, it is unfortunate that it got to the stage where I didn't feel part of a team effort. When you feel it isn't one for all and all for one any more, it makes things difficult.

Overall I felt that I was drifting at Ducati, that I was overstaying my welcome and that it would be wise under the circumstances to move on as quickly as I could. I was also worried that if Troy Bayliss and Lanzi, a brilliant Italian, were available then there may no longer be room for me. I felt as if I was just seeing out my contract. It didn't faze me too much, but it made me determined to go out fighting. And in my last race for them at Magny-Cours, the scene of my great triumph the year before, I had a huge battle with Karl Muggeridge, my old Aussie foe, and ended up winning, and then coming third in the second leg.

Despite all the problems I had encountered, I nearly pipped Haga for third place in the championship. It gave me a real boost to think how close I came to a top-three finale. I reasoned that I hadn't been riding all that badly and if I could finish that well in the title chase, despite my horrific season, I must have been doing something right. But if Ducati didn't want to renew my contract, well, so be it.

I didn't know for sure at this point that I no longer had a job with Ducati, despite the rumours that Bayliss was coming back from MotoGP and Lanzi was in the frame. But, astonishingly, and without my suspecting anything, a few races before the end, Tardozzi had been up the paddock talking about me to the Dutch owners of the Ten Kate Honda team. I was shocked when Davide told me Ten Kate were interested in me, even before I knew that I wasn't going to stay on at Ducati. That's how tough and surprising this business can be. However, I didn't fall out with him and, in truth, he did me a massive favour. I found out afterwards that he had given me a glowing reference and had praised my personality and attitude.

But moving to the Ten Kate team depended on whether their rider Chris Vermeulen, as rumours suggested, was going to switch to MotoGP. Even so, just to make sure the team knew how keen I was to join them, Roger Burnett arranged a meeting with them in Holland. It was clear that this was our only chance, slim though it was, to hold onto a place on the WSB grid. All the other teams had signed up their riders, and Vermeulen's move seemed to have been stalled. The only other options were to return to British Superbikes with my old friend and sponsor John Jones and his HM Plant–Honda team, or to link up with my mate Neil Hodgson in America for the stateside championship, a move which would have been supported and encouraged by Ducati. But I wasn't, despite John Jones's eagerness to recruit me, ready to make what I felt would be a step backwards onto the BSB stage. Nor was I all that eager to cross the Atlantic. Sure, the money would have been better and I'd have had a great team-mate in Hodgson, not to mention a lot of fun with all the sun, glamour and beaches. But no: I wanted to complete some unfinished business in WSB. I wanted that title back. And I wanted it badly. It was this drive and motivation that excited Ten Kate and convinced them that I would be just the guy to take over where Vermeulen left off.

Eventually, Chris did decide to opt out when Suzuki moved for him, and owners and cousins, Gerrit and Ronald Ten Kate, invited Roger and me to Holland to clear up the finer details of my new deal. There were no differences in terms of money or conditions, and it was all done amicably and quickly. When we were wrapping up the meeting, Ronald revealed that one of the factors that convinced them to take me on was my never-say-die spirit. 'We admired how hard you fought for that podium place, for yourself and the team, in that last race after such a difficult year,' he said. I was grateful that they had recognised my strength and determination in the face of adversity.

It was a great relief and a tremendous lift because I knew that Honda, who had a major say in rider move-ment to satellite teams, were interested in three mega names currently unsettled in MotoGP: Max Biaggi, Alex Barros and Troy Bayliss. But to my eternal gratitude Ten Kate argued that their preference was for me and insisted that the Japanese should follow Gerrit's and Ronald's instincts and wishes.

As I said, I would have been paid more to go to AMA in America, but WSB was where I most wanted to be and the thought that I might miss out was too awful to contemplate. If I'd been, say, thirty and an ex-world champion with a career end looming, looking to wind down, then I might have been tempted by AMA. But I really felt that at that moment in my life I needed to make as big an effort as I could to be world champion for a second time.

I wasn't really in a strong bargaining position with Ten Kate so I couldn't haggle for a better deal during that first tentative meeting with the cousins. I would have done anything to get to ride and that's what I wanted to get across to them. To tell the truth, I found myself in a far better situation with Ten Kate Honda than I had at Ducati – financially as well as professionally. The basic pay was roughly the same, but where Ducati retained the rights to advertising space on my helmets, boots, leathers and gloves, Ten Kate handed those opportunities for extra revenue over to me.

They are a small but brilliantly organised and determined team, and a semi-works set-up to rival the full-blown works boys. It gives the garage a terrific buzz; it's like the underdogs biting back.

My only worry was that I had never raced a four-stroke before. My entire Superbike career had been on twin-cylinder bikes. I wondered how I would adapt to the change with the Honda; its characteristics were so different to what I had grown used to. The Ten Kate people were also curious to see how I would cope, but I assured them that I would put in the effort to get to grips with the new bike. I stressed that I would give it 110 per cent, as I always aim to do, to overcome any doubts they might have had.

After we shook hands on the deal at the Ten Kate factory in Holland and I was guaranteed another year in WSB, I resolved to do everything I could to win the championship, for them as much as for me. I was confident that I had impressed them and Roger and I enjoyed a celebration beer – bought by me – at Amsterdam's Schiphol airport. We headed home excited and relieved that I wouldn't have to agonise through a spell of unemployment. I had got exactly what I wanted.

During the build-up to my departure from Ducati and my signing for Ten Kate there had been an annoying catalogue of misunderstandings from certain sections of the press of the difficulties I had undergone with the Italian team. This ranged from suggestions that I was a one-season wonder to insinuations that I wouldn't be able to cope with the change from twin- to four-stroke machinery at Honda. It was as if my career was in freefall. However, this only fired me up even more and made me determined to prove my critics wrong.

I have to confess the first couple of tests were really difficult and I needed to overcome some major problems quickly. The first time I ever rode the bike was at Valencia in the damp and that was a real eye-opener. It was a nightmare to ride without traction control having got used to it on the Ducati. My feet were off the pegs everywhere, I was biting the screen on every corner and I was in a right mess. It felt odd and unfamiliar, as if I'd borrowed somebody else's bike. It didn't feel like mine at all. I realised that it was going to take a lot of hard work to get the bike and me working as one.

I took a New Year's break with the family in Euro Disney and made sure I chilled out and got my head clear for what was going to be a tough task. Then, at the next two test sessions, with a few bits and pieces put on the Honda and an injection of boldness from me, it all started coming together. The bike was doing about 90 per cent of what I wanted it to do, my confidence began to pick up and my lap times started tumbling down. Suddenly, I felt we were travelling in the right direction.

The team were fantastic: unhurried, ice cool and not the least bit panicky. They worked hard to give me what I needed and over each test session I gained the confidence to take the bike to the edge and run it at competitive rates. Sure, there was still a shortage of experience that could put me at a disadvantage as I headed towards the first 2006 season race in Qatar, but I accepted the situation and made the best of it. My mood and motivation were high and I was prepared to make up for the shortfall with sheer balls and determination. However close I had to get to the threshold and whatever risks I took were necessary, if not to be a winner right away then to be a front-runner.

Of course, there was also the small matter of the opposition – the strongest, most talented line-up ever in WSB. Cross-over MotoGP rider Alex Barros, who'd had plenty of wins and had beaten Valentino Rossi, Rolfo, Bayliss and Xaus; Corser, the reigning WSB champ, stunningly fast and stronger than ever on the Suzuki; Haga, as well, on a much better Yamaha was always a considerable threat. All men to beat. Any one of them had the potential to be a winner, something I was all too aware of as I headed for Qatar. But I never imagined that I was destined for a dream start in this new phase of my career.

I had, incidentally, a scare that I might have contracted scarlet fever before the season started. I was really sick and I had never felt so ill in my life. A Harley Street doctor blitzed me with some really powerful antibiotics and warned me that if the tablets didn't work then it was more than likely I had scarlet fever. I was really scared. Thankfully, however, it just turned out to be a really heavy bout of 'flu that had downed me.

By the time I got to the Middle East, I was in good shape again, feeling really fit and on top of my game. I was also looking forward to the chance to show that I was capable of beating some established MotoGP guys, the so-called elite class of motorbike racing, and ram some of the nastier comments back down the throats of my critics.

I qualified on the front row, but during the race I got caught out with my unfamiliarity with the CBR1000RR. I got off to the worst possible start off the line. The Honda is a specialised sort of starter, you have to be careful not to rev it over the 8,000 mark or the clutch plays up. You have to watch four lights on the dashboard under the bubble to make sure they're all synchronised, while at the same time keeping an eye on the gantry lights that signal the start. And all this amid the noise, chaos, excitement, adrenalin flow and anticipation.

Disastrously, I got a bit distracted trying to keep one eye on the start lights and the other one on the bike, and by the time I'd got going I was down to fourteenth with one hell of a battle facing me to get up with the leaders, who had opened up a gap of four or five seconds ahead of me. That's a massive gap to shut down, and I was going to be playing an agonising game of catch-up with some really quick riders on superb machines. I had to make up at least half a second a lap. Amazingly, I did and that gave me a huge boost of confidence because it meant I was faster than the front men. I caught up with them for third place by the last lap. Then I had a massive stroke of luck. Yukio Kagayama and Nori Haga took each other out yards from the finish line, and I inherited victory.

Of course, it was a fantastically fortunate break for me — but, honestly, I rated it as my best performance ever. And that view was backed up by the critics, who all at once were eager to sing my praises rather than write me off as a no-hoper. I can't explain how satisfied I felt.

I loved reading afterwards in *Motorcycle News*: 'With no previous experience of a four-cylinder superbike, Toseland was expected to take a few races to get up to speed on his Fireblade, but he showed the grit and passion that won him the title in 2004.' It was written under the headline: 'BRIT EXCEEDS EXPECTATION TO TAKE FIRST RACE WIN IN QATAR'.

I rode as hard as I could and was ruthless. I made a critical and crucial move on Corser on the brakes, nearly barging him off, and I confessed to the press afterwards: 'I made a naughty pass on Troy – but I was committed to the corner.' When Haga and Kagayama went down in front of me I could have cheered. They handed me my first win since Silverstone in 2005, but I had worked bloody hard and taken a lot of risks to get back into contention after my appalling start. The no-hoper was a returnee to the big game as a serious challenger, especially to the champion and the MotoGP come-overs, who were all expected to leave me trailing.

The second race was no less exciting. A thrilling showdown in which I lost out by the almost immeasurable margin of 1.5cm, about a thousandth of a second, to Haga for a third place photo-finish that robbed me of the top spot in the championship chase. I put a heavy move on Haga when I was sideways on in the final turn and almost shoved him off, but, with no traction control to help, my wheels were spinning and losing grip and he got a better drive out of the corner and beat me to the line by the tiniest of margins. Fourth. But I had registered my return to the top end of WSB with an impressive haul at Qatar, and a picture of my dogged determination and willingness to take chances was now firmly logged in the minds of my critics and the riders I was going to be up against for the rest of the season.

Team chief Ronald Ten Kate, whose team had won ten WSB races and four World Supersport titles, told the press: 'Your Englishman is some racer! In the first race he was so far back that most riders would have given up or even pulled in with some stupid excuse – but not James ...

'Usually, our team progresses a lot during the season, so to win the first race makes me very happy.'

I had barely got a mention in the specialist motorcycle race press throughout the winter. It was all Corser, Barros, Biaggi, Haga and Bayliss, and no Toseland. But my Qatar showing quickly put that right. It was lovely. I headed for Australia and Phillip Island – with my mum in tow as a fiftieth birthday present – in high hopes and full of confidence for round two. The team was delighted, and it showed. They realised that the Toseland name was back in the frame. And, what's more, I was still learning the bike.

I had never been on the podium at Phillip Island. There always seemed to be something going wrong to keep me out of the top three even though I was good and quick there; a wrong tyre being put on, rain or being knocked off had dropped me out of it. I was determined to put things right this time round and I got off to a fantastic start with a third place on the front row of the grid. In race one, I got a good start but Bayliss cleared off to a four second or so lead, and I managed third. In the second leg, I was runner-up, ahead of Barros, to winner Corser – and that gave me enough points to close to within one point of title pacemaker Bayliss with his full-blown works Ducati.

I was still struggling to master the vagaries of a bike without traction control, with total reliance on my ability and feel for the throttle, and yet was managing to put together some impressive rides. Then we were told that Japan had promised to give us the extra boost of technology and infuse some MotoGP engineering expertise into our WSB effort. Traction control was on its way! At long last we would have the same benefits as Ducati, Suzuki, Kawasaki and Yamaha, who all ran with the system.

After my double podium down under, I told the media that I was really happy with how fast we were. After only four races, I was just one point off the lead. Bayliss was quick, and he knew his bike very well, better than I knew mine. But I still ended up on the podium alongside him and Barros. I felt comfortable and competitive with them and I am not intimidated by any of them. Both the Honda and I are capable of beating them.

As one of my heavier critics, *Motorcycle News*, recently affirmed in a headline: 'THE OLD TOSELAND IS BACK.'

Epilogue

STAYING POWER

I have always maintained that the one person you cannot lie to is yourself; sure, you can fool yourself and those around you, but deep down you cannot deceive yourself.

When I look back at where I am now and where I came from, I am astounded and proud. My dreams had plenty of reason to falter and fade away, but I am hugely appreciative of all the people, especially my mum, who believed in me and helped me believe in myself. Being a world champion at any sport is clearly an outstanding achievement. Because of the way I was brought up, to be humble in success and grateful for the genuine concerns of others, it is not difficult for me to remind myself that without the encouragement of those you respect and who love you, the chances of attainment are very slim indeed. I don't want to sound like a Hollywood Oscar winner making a soppy tribute to everybody and his uncle, but I really do have to thank my mum, Jane, for those early lessons. Her constant reminders throughout my teens and early twenties made me the man I am now and, hopefully, the rounded person she always hoped I would be.

She did that and a lot more. A hell of a lot more.

My peaceful new home is in Ramsey, a little fishing harbour in the Isle of Man, just a few miles from the capital Douglas. I sit there among the beautiful scenery and picture the most remarkable and magical year of my life, the 2004 race season when I was crowned World

Superbike champion. I could not have done it without the crucial help of a tremendous team of people backing me. However, without wanting to give the impression that I am arrogant or egotistic, it was my own skill and effort that helped me beat the best Superbike riders in the world to become the champion. Nobody can take that away from me, whatever happens in the future. The satisfaction I get from that is unique and indescribable. My name is on the trophy, it is in the record books for all time and it stands as a testimonial of everything I have learned – personal sacrifice, determination, triumph over self-doubt at times, and a willingness to listen to the advice and counsel of others who know better. Above all, it is a tribute to people who kept faith in my ability when, at times, it may have seemed to be wavering.

I have always maintained that the one person you cannot lie to is yourself: sure, you can fool yourself and those around you, but deep down you cannot deceive yourself. That is one of my strengths. I have never tried to kid myself that I am better or worse than I am. If you fall for falsehoods, persuaded by your own short-sightedness, you are sure to get your comeuppance. And what could be more embarrassing than that? Down to earth is where my mum says the most honest people dwell. And that's exactly where I began and will stay whatever further achievements come my way. I could never see myself in the same light that firm and committed fans, or even outsiders, see me.

Oddly, a question that seems to crop up regularly is: do you ever wish you were a bit more arrogant so that you could get even more, and demand deeper respect, out of being the world champion? The answer I will always make to that query is straightforward and, I trust, a fair and completely frank reflection of my personality: I honestly do not know how to change. I am who I am. No more. No less. I guess I am like everybody else who, by nature and normal evolution, seems to have character changes about every ten years, but nothing spectacular or life-changing. And after all, I am still young, so there's a long way to go.

I see, hear or read interviews I did years ago where I draw attention to myself winning and realise that I was saying virtually what I was told or advised to say. All my answers had to be politically correct, rather than having my own opinion. Nowadays, the difference is that I say what I am thinking in as balanced a fashion as I can manage. I still err on the safe side of so-called political correctness, without grovelling to anybody or any organisation, but now I make sure it is my own opinion I am getting across, and not the prompting from somebody else with an agenda. I feel that I am a lot more positive in what I say; I certainly think a lot about the answers I am going to give before I open my mouth.

I am probably the most critical judge of my character and, without sounding paranoid, I look hard at myself all the time and strive to learn the lessons from other people's reactions. For example, when I am sitting at home with my family and I come out and say something which isn't necessarily what I would actually want to say, maybe because I hadn't thought it out thoroughly enough, it either sounds immodest or not right. It's only because of the emotions that are going through my head that the delivery gets fogged and I sound arrogant and self-centred, but I always find myself looking at my brother or my mum and seeing a reaction that says without words: Ooooh, that's a bit over the top – cocky bugger! Then I twig right away and learn from the lesson. After all, my brother and my mum have known me since I was a baby and I can only judge my attitude now on conversations I have with them, and their responses. If all of a sudden you don't have anything in common with the family that has nurtured and cherished you with selfless affection and protection all your life, you must know there is something sadly wrong.

I know there are lots of achievers – famous, moderately famous, local heroes hardly known outside their immediate environment, and champions even – who don't get recognised to the level that they are worthy of. But, honestly, I don't get the least bit miffed if I am not immediately the name or face that springs to mind when I am introduced into company or am walking down the street.

People who only view you from a distance can often get the wrong impression. Maybe that is why I don't let people get too close and why I want to do my best to ensure that the correct picture of me is being formed. I know one thing for sure: my concerns about character perception all stem back to my childhood. What's more, when I go right back to the start, there is so much that people don't know – that I didn't know before I started to write this book – and that I still to this day find hard to relive without wondering how I ever found the motivation to survive.

My Ducati backers were fabulous and gave me a grand opportunity to achieve all my ambitions; the focus and motivation had to come from myself; but it took the wide-eyed appreciation of one of my little nephews to bring something else to the equation. OK, I had the trophy, the adulation and the title of World Champion, but it took that wee fellow saying, 'You must be somebody special now?' to make me realise the simplicity of my achievement. Sometimes it takes a kid's innocent remark to re-tune you to reality.

JAMES TOSELAND STATISTICS

James Toseland All Time Statistics

2005 Season Team Ducati Xerox
Bike Ducati
Race Number 1

Year		Poles	Races	Podiums	Wins	2nd pl.	3rd pl.	Fast l.	Titles
All times	Superbike	1	108	27	5	12	10		1
All times	Supersport		17						

	Year		Poles	Races	Podiums	Wins	2nd pl.	3rd pl.	Fast l.	Ch. pos.
7	2005	Superbike		12	3	1		2		5th
6	2004	Superbike		22	14	3	9	2		1st
5	2003	Superbike	1	24	9	1	3	5		3rd
4	2002	Superbike		26	1			1		7th
3	2001	Superbike		24						13th
2	1999	Supersport		–						11th
1	1998	Supersport		–						19th

*Statistics correct at time of print.

All Time Player Statistics

	Rider	Poles	Races	Podiums	Wins	2nd pl.	3rd pl.	Fast l.	Ch. pos.
1	Fogarty Carl	21	219	109	59	33	17	47	4
2	Edwards Colin	15	175	75	31	24	20	23	2
3	Corser Troy	32	215	91	29	32	30	38	1
4	Polen Doug	17	79	40	27	8	5	17	2
5	Roche Raymond	9	95	57	23	23	11	25	1
6	Bayliss Troy	7	76	46	22	18	6	13	1
7	Chili Pierfrancesco	10	249	61	17	18	26	29	
8	Haga Noriyuki	2	144	41	17	11	13	20	
9	Falappa Giancarlo	8	106	30	16	6	8	11	
10	Hodgson Neil	16	147	41	16	15	10	14	1
11	Kocinski John	6	48	29	14	7	8	11	1
12	Russell Scott	8	117	39	14	17	8	8	1
13	Slight Aaron	8	229	87	13	42	32	26	
14	Laconi Régis	7	81	26	11	7	8	10	
15	Mertens Stephane	3	154	45	11	15	19	8	
16	Pirovano Fabrizio		183	47	10	14	23	13	
17	Xaus Ruben	1	77	31	9	12	10	11	
18	Gobert Anthony	2	57	16	8	3	5	2	
19	Merkel Fred	4	114	24	8	6	10	7	2
20	Bostrom Ben	2	93	17	7	4	6	5	
21	Tardozzi Davide	2	75	11	5	2	4	2	

#	Name								
22	Toseland James	1	108	27	5	12	10		1
23	Vermeulen Chris		34	15	5	8	2	5	
24	Phillis Rob	3	105	27	4	13	10	6	
25	Doohan Michael	1	4	3	3			1	
26	Tamada Makoto	1	6	4	3	1		3	
27	Yanagawa Akira	2	118	23	3	9	11	6	
28	Byrne Shane		6	2	2			1	
29	Chandler Doug	1	14	5	2		3	1	
30	Dowson Michael	1	14	6	2	3	1	2	

All Time Manufacturer Statistics

	Manufacturer	Poles	Races	Podiums	Wins	2nd pl.	3rd pl.	Fast l.	Ch. wins
1	Ducati	127	–	600	239	200	161	230	13
2	Honda	34	–	268	81	94	93	79	4
3	Kawasaki	18	–	160	34	58	68	36	
4	Yamaha	10	–	127	34	38	55	32	
5	Suzuki	9	–	61	15	18	28	26	
6	Bimota	4	–	22	11	7	4	5	
7	Aprilia	8	–	26	8	6	12	12	
8	Benelli		–						
9	MV Agusta		–						
10	Petronas	2	–	2		1	1		

World Championship Results

	Poles	Races	Podiums	Wins	2nd	3rd	Fast l.	Position
1998 Supersport								
1 Pirovano Fabrizio	1	–	7	5	1	1	3	1st
2 Guareschi Vittoriano	3	–	6	1	2	3	1	2nd
3 Chambon Stephane	1	–	5	1	3	1	1	3rd
4 Casoli Paolo	2	–	2	2				4th
5 Meregalli Massimo		–	2		1	1		5th
6 Migliorati Cristiano	1	–	2		1	1	2	6th
7 Riba Pere	2	–	2		1	1	2	7th
8 Zeelenberg Wilco		–	2					8th
9 Bussei Giovanni		–						9th
10 Ulm Robert		–						10th
11 Lucchiari Mauro		–	2		1			11th
12 Briguet Yves		–	1			1	1	12th
13 Charpentier Sébastien		–	1	1				13th
14 Fiorillo Giuseppe		–						14th
15 Risitano Marco		–						15th
16 Teneggi Roberto		–						16th
17 Teuchert Jörg		–						17th
18 Mariottini Camillo		–						18th
19 Toseland James		–						19th
20 Pridmore Jason		–						20th

World Championship Results *continued*

1999 Supersport

	Poles	Races	Podiums	Wins	2nd	3rd	Fast l.	Position
1 Chambon Stephane	3	–	5	2	2	1	2	1st
2 MacPherson Iain	2	–	5	3	1	1	3	2nd
3 Bontempi Piergiorgio	1	–	3	1	1	1	1	3rd
4 Teuchert Jorg	1	–	3	2		1		4th
5 Xaus Ruben	2	–	5	1	3	1		5th
6 Kellner Christian		–	1		1		1	6th
7 Pirovano Fabrizio		–	2		1			7th
8 Migliorati Cristiano		–	2			1		8th
9 Zeelenberg Wilco		–	2	1		1		9th
10 Costes William		–	1			1		10th
11 Toseland James		–						11th
12 Meregalli Massimo	1	–	1			1	1	12th
13 Riba Pere		–	1			1	1	13th
14 Casoli Paolo	1	–	2		1	1	1	14th
15 Cogan Christophe		–						15th
16 Whitham James		–	1	1			1	16th
17 Briguet Yves		–						17th
18 Iannuzzo Vittorio		–						18th
19 Charpentier Sébastien		–						19th
20 Harris Dan		–						20th

	Poles	Races	Podiums	Wins	2nd	3rd	Fast l.	Position
2001 World Superbike								
1 Bayliss Troy	2	24	15	6	6	3	3	1st
2 Edwards Colin		25	12	4	3	5	4	2nd
3 Bostrom Ben	2	25	9	6	1	2	3	3rd
4 Corser Troy	3	25	10	2	3	5	4	4th
5 Hodgson Neil	4	25	7	1	5	1	1	5th
6 Xaus Ruben		25	6	2	4		4	6th
7 Chili Pierfrancesco		25	2	1	1		2	7th
8 Okada Tadayuki		25	3		1	2		8th
9 Yanagawa Akira		23	2			2		9th
10 Lavilla Gregorio		25	2			2		10th
11 Laconi Régis		25	1	1				11th
12 Chambon Stephane		25						12th
13 Toseland James		24						13th
14 Izutsu Hitoyasu		9	2		1	1		14th
15 Tamada Makoto	1	2	2	2			2	15th
16 Parkes Broc		22						16th
17 Martin Steve		25						17th
18 Bussei Giovanni		25						18th
19 Pedercini Lucio		25						19th
20 Ulm Robert								

257

	Poles	Races	Podiums	Wins	2nd	3rd	Fast l.	Position
2002 World Superbike								
1 Edwards Colin	5	26	25	11	10	4	8	1st
2 Bayliss Troy	4	26	22	14	7	1	9	2nd
3 Hodgson Neil	3	26	9		2	7	1	3rd
4 Haga Noriyuki	1	26	7		3	4	4	4th
5 Bostrom Ben		26	1			1	1	5th
6 Xaus Ruben		26	10		2	8	2	6th
7 Toseland James		26	1			1		7th
8 Chili Pierfrancesco		24	1		1			8th
9 Walker Chris		26						9th
10 Lavilla Gregorio		24						10th
11 Parkes Broc		25						11th
12 Borja Juan Bautista		22						12th
13 Pedercini Lucio		26						13th
14 Izutsu Hitoyasu		14						14th
15 Borciani Marco		26						15th
16 Martin Steve		23						16th
17 Bostrom Eric		8						17th
18 Tamada Makoto		2	2	1	1		1	18th
19 Sanchini Mauro		26						19th
20 Antonello Alessandro		26						20th

	Poles	Races	Podiums	Wins	2nd	3rd	Fast l.	Position
2003 World Superbike								
1 Hodgson Neil	6	24	20	13	7		10	1st
2 Xaus Ruben	1	24	15	7	6	2	5	2nd
3 Toseland James	1	24	9	1	3	5		3rd
4 Laconi Regis	1	24	5		3	2	2	4th
5 Lavilla Gregorio		24	7		3	4	3	5th
6 Walker Chris		24	6			6		6th
7. Chili Pierfrancesco	1	24	7	1	1	5	2	7th
8 Martin Steve		24						8th
9 Pedercini Lucio		24						9th
10 Borciani Marco		24						10th
11 Sanchini Mauro		24						11th
12 Corser Troy		24						12th
13 Borja Juan Bautista		22						13th
14 Clementi Ivan		24						14th
15 Bussei Giovanni		16						15th
16 Byrne Shane		2	2	2			1	16th
17 Reynolds John	1	6	1		1		1	17th
18 Iannuzzo Vittorio		8						18th
19 Gramigni Alex		14						19th
20 Kagayama Yukio		4						20th

The 2004 Season

11/02/2004	Winter Test
29/02/2004	Valencia
28/03/2004	Phillip Island
18/04/2004	Misano Adriatico
16/05/2004	Monza
30/05/2004	Oschersleben
13/06/2004	Silverstone
11/07/2004	Laguna Seca
01/08/2004	Brands Hatch
05/09/2004	Assen
26/09/2004	Imola
03/10/2004	Magny-Cours

Championship Results

	Poles	Races	Podiums	Wins	2nd	3rd	Fast L.	Position
1 Toseland James		22	14	3	9	2		1st
2 Laconi Régis	5	22	14	7	2	5	6	2nd
3 Haga Noriyuki		22	9	6	2	1	7	3rd
4 Vermeulen Chris		22	9	4	4	1	3	4th
5 Chili Pierfrancesco	1	22	9	4	4	4	3	5th
6 McCoy Garry		22	3	1	1	2	2	6th
7 Martin Steve	3	22	5			5	1	7th
8 Haslam Leon		22	1			1		8th
9 Corser Troy	2	22	1		1			9th
10 Borciani Marco		22						10th
11 Walker Chris		22	1			1		11th
12 Clementi Ivan		21						12th
13 Sanchini Mauro		17						13th
14 Nannelli Gianluca		22						14th
15 Bontempi Piergiorgio		22						15th
16 Pedercini Lucio		21						16th
17 Fuertes Sergio		18						17th
18 Gimbert Sebastien		4						18th
19 Ellison James		4						19th
20 Nowland Warwick		18						20th

2004 Season Winter Test

	Riders	Laps	Times		Riders	Laps	Times
1	Laconi Régis	156	1'35.393	13	Chili Pierfrancesco	96	1'37.343
2	Martin Steve	117	1'35.574	14	McCoy Garry	128	1'37.585
3	Toseland James	190	1'36.162	15	Pedercini Lucio	146	1'37.674
4	Haslam Leon	151	1'36.201	16	Schulten Michael	82	1'37.821
5	Borciani Marco	150	1'36.303	17	Nannelli Gianluca	34	1'37.840
6	Corser Troy	91	1'36.310	18	Bontempi Piergiorgio	135	1'38.512
7	Haga Noriyuki	101	1'36.676	19	De Matteis Giancarlo	98	1'38.568
8	Vermeulen Chris	125	1'36.907	20	Praia Miguel	145	1'39.033
9	Fuertes Sergio	87	1'37.023	21	Oelschlager Jurgen	100	1'39.148
10	Clementi Ivan	124	1'37.186	22	Velini Alessio	137	1'39.276
11	Sanchini Mauro	129	1'37.281	23	Nowland Warwick	166	1'39.303
12	Walker Chris	114	1'37.287	24	Saiger Horst	191	1'39.867

VALENCIA 29/02/2004

Valencia

Name: RICARDO TORMO
Circuit length: 4005 m
Pole position: Right
Maximum slope: down 5.33%–up 3.58%

Corners left: 9 **Right:** 5
Corner radius: min. 30 m–max. 250 m
Finish line length: 876 m

Best lap	2003	Hodgson Neil	Ducati 1'34.633
Superpole record	2002	Bayliss Troy	Ducati 1'34.814
Race record	2003	Hodgson Neil	Ducati 1'35.007

Riders	Teams	Bikes	Laps	Times
SUNDAY 12.00 RACE 1				
1 Toseland James	Ducati Fila	Ducati 999 F04	23	42'39.266
2 Chili Pierfrancesco	PSG – 1 Corse	Ducati 999 RS	23	42'43.964
3 Walker Chris	Foggy PETRONAS Racing	Petronas FP1	23	43'01.375
4 Borciani Marco	D.F.Xtreme Sterilgarda	Ducati 999 RS	23	43'32.570
5 Haslam Leon	Renegade Ducati	Ducati 999 RS	23	43'41.552
SUNDAY 15.30 RACE 2				
1 Haga Noriyuki	Renegade Ducati	Ducati 999 RS	23	37'32.364
2 Toseland James	Ducati Fila	Ducati 999 F04	23	37'34.133
3 Martin Steve	D.F.Xtreme Sterilgarda	Ducati 999 RS	23	37'42.385
4 Chili Pierfrancesco	PSG – 1 Corse	Ducati 999 RS	23	37'42.502
5 Vermeulen Chris	Ten Kate Honda	Honda CBR 1000RR	23	37'49.431

PHILLIP ISLAND 28/03/2004

Phillip Island

Name: PHILLIP ISLAND
Circuit length: 4445 m
Pole position: Left
Maximum slope: 57 m

Corners left: 7 Right: 3
Corner radius: min. 23 m–max. 207 m
Finish line length: 835 m

Best lap	1999	Corser Troy	Ducati 1'32.193
Superpole record	1999	Corser Troy	Ducati 1'32.193
Race record	1999	Corser Troy	Ducati 1'33.019

Riders	Teams	Bikes	Laps	Times
SUNDAY 12.00 RACE 1				
1 Laconi Régis	Ducati Fila	Ducati 999 F04	22	35'04.598
2 Vermeulen Chris	Ten Kate Honda	Honda CBR 1000RR	22	35'11.743
3 Toseland James	Ducati Fila	Ducati 999 F04	22	35'12.134
4 Martin Steve	D.F.Xtreme Sterilgarda	Ducati 999 RS	22	35'12.215
5 McCoy Garry	XEROX – Ducati Nortel Net.	Ducati 999 RS	22	35'12.406
SUNDAY 15.30 RACE 2				
1 McCoy Garry	XEROX – Ducati Nortel Net.	Ducati 999 RS	22	35'10.023
2 Vermeulen Chris	Ten Kate Honda	Honda CBR 1000RR	22	35'14.974
3 Chili Pierfrancesco	PSG – 1 Corse	Ducati 998 RS	22	35'16.462
4 Borciani Marco	D.F.Xtreme Sterilgarda	Ducati 999 RS	22	35'18.852
5 Corser Troy	Foggy PETRONAS Racing	Petronas FP1	22	35'21.847

MISANO ADRIATICO 18/04/2004

Misano Adriatico

Name: SANTA MONICA
Circuit length: 4060 m
Pole position: Left
Maximum slope: 1.5%

Corners left: 4 **Right:** 4
Corner radius: min. 28 m–max. 74 m
Finish line length: 510 m

Best lap	2002	Baylis Troy	Ducati 1'33.525
Superpole record	2002	Baylis Troy	Ducati 1'33.525
Race record	2002	Baylis Troy	Ducati 1'34.913

	Riders	Teams	Bikes	Laps	Times
SUNDAY 12.00 RACE 1					
1	Laconi Régis	Ducati Fila	Ducati 999 F04	17	28'18.586
2	Corser Troy	Foggy PETRONAS Racing	Petronas FP1	17	28'20.530
3	Chili Pierfrancesco	PSG – 1 Corse	Ducati 998 RS	17	28'26.045
4	Haga Noriyuki	Renegade Ducati	Ducati 999 RS	17	28'28.314
5	Vermeulen Chris	Ten Kate Honda	Honda CBR 1000RR	17	28'30.896
SUNDAY 15.30 RACE 2					
1	Chili Pierfrancesco	PSG – 1 Corse	Ducati 998 RS	25	44'29.370
2	Laconi Régis	Ducati Fila	Ducati 999 F04	25	44'30.854
3	Martin Steve	D.F.Xtreme Sterilgarda	Ducati 999 RS	25	45'01.629
4	Li Naga Noriyuki	Renegade Ducati	Ducati 999 RS	25	45'07.458
5	Haslam Leon	Renegade Ducati	Ducati 999 RS	25	45'10.401
(Toseland 6th)					

MONZA 16/05/2004

Monza

Name: AUTODROMO NAZIONALE
Circuit length: 5793 m
Pole position: Left
Maximum slope: 2.4% + 1.7%

Corners left: 5 Right: 8
Corner radius: min. 12.50 m – max. 610.00 m
Finish line length: 1195 m

Best lap	2003	Hodgson Neil	Ducati 1'46.981
Superpole record	2003	Hodgson Neil	Ducati 1'46.981
Race record	2002	Bayliss Troy	Ducati 1'47.434

Riders	Teams	Bikes	Laps	Times
SUNDAY 12.00 RACE 1				
1 Laconi Régis	Ducati Fila	Ducati 999 F04	18	32'53.859
2 Toseland James	Ducati Fila	Ducati 999 F04	18	33'03.659
3 McCoy Garry	XEROX – Ducati Norte! Net.	Ducati 999 RS	18	33'05.750
4 Vermeulen Chris	Ten Kate Honda	Honda CBR 1000RR	18	33'27.914
5 Haslam Leon	Renegade Ducati	Ducati 999 RS	18	33'31.880
SUNDAY 15.30 RACE 2				
1 Laconi Régis	Ducati Fila	Ducati 999 F04	18	32'48.901
2 Toseland James	Ducati Fila	Ducati 999 F04	18	33'07.182
3 McCoy Garry	XEROX – Ducati Nortel Net.	Ducati 999 RS	18	33'08.304
4 Haslam Leon	Renegade Ducati	Ducati 999 RS	18	33'23.512
5 Corser Troy	Foggy PETRONAS Racing	Petronas FP1	18	33'29.566

OSCHERSLEBEN 30/05/2004

Oschersleben

Name: OSCHERSLEBEN
Circuit length: 3667 m
Pole position: Right
Maximum slope: 2.50%

Corners left: 7 **Right:** 7
Corner radius: min. 44 m–max. 70 m
Finish line length: 680 m

Best lap	2002	Hodgson Neil	Ducati 1'26.502
Superpole record	2002	Hodgson Neil	Ducati 1'26.502
Race record	2002	Edwards Collin	Honda 1'26.549

	Riders	Teams	Bikes	Laps	Times
SUNDAY 12.00 RACE 1					
1	Haga Noriyuki	Renegade Ducati	Ducati 999 RS	28	41'49.906
2	Toseland James	Ducati Fila	Ducati 999 F04	28	41'55.070
3	Chili Pierfrancesco	PSG – 1 Corse	Ducati 998 RS	28	41'55.229
4	Corser Troy	Foggy PETRONAS Racing	Petronas FP1	28	42'02.930
5	Martin Steve	D.F.Xtreme Sterilgarda	Ducati 999 RS	28	42'10.088
SUNDAY 15.30 RACE 2					
1	Laconi Régis	Ducati Fila	Ducati 999 F04	28	41'50.459
2	Toseland James	Ducati Fila	Ducati 999 F04	28	42'12.008
3	Haslam Leon	Renegade Ducati	Ducati 999 RS	28	42'15.144
4	McCoy Garry	XEROX – Ducati Nortel Net.	Ducati 999 RS	28	42'17.872
5	Nannelli Gianluca	Pedercini	Ducati 998 RS	28	42'21.080

SILVERSTONE 13/06/2004

Silverstone

Name: SILVERSTONE
Circuit length: 3561 m
Pole position: Right

Corners left: 5 Right: 7
Finish line length: 491 m

			Bikes
Best lap	2005	Kagayama Yukio	Suzuki 1'26.679
Superpole record	2005	Kagayama Yukio	Suzuki 1'26.679
Race record	2005	Laconi Régis	Ducati 1'27.130

	Riders	Teams	Bikes	Laps	Times
SUNDAY 12.00 RACE 1					
1	Haga Noriyuki	Renegade Ducati	Ducati 999 RS	20	38'43.657
2	Vermeulen Chris	Ten Kate Honda	Honda CBR 1000RR	20	38'43.807
3	Chili Pierfrancesco	PSG – 1 Corse	Ducati 998 RS	20	38'50.240
4	McCoy Garry	XEROX – Ducati Nortel Net.	Ducati 999 RS	20	3910.920
5	Haslam Leon	Renegade Ducati	Ducati 999 RS	20	39'11.237
SUNDAY 15.30 RACE 2					
1	Vermeulen Chris	Ten Kate Honda	Honda CBR 1000RR	20	38'35.608
2	Haga Noriyuki	Renegade Ducati	Ducati 999 RS	20	38'35.836
3	Laconi Régis	Ducati Fila	Ducati 999 F04	20	38'41.763
4	Haslam Leon	Renegade Ducati	Ducati 999 RS	20	38'56.503
5	Toseland James	Ducati Fila	Ducati 999 F04	20	39'03.112

LAGUNA SECA 11/07/2004

Laguna Seca

Name: LAGUNA SECA
Circuit length: 3610 m
Pole position: Right
Maximum slope: downward 30%

Corners left: 6 **Right:** 4
Corner radius: min. 14 m–max. 158 m
Finish line length: 300 m

Best lap	2002	Bayliss Troy		Ducati 1'24.833
Superpole record	2002	Edwards Collin		Honda 1'24.888
Race record	2002	Haga Noriyuki		Aprilia 1'25.475

Riders	Teams	Bikes	Laps	Times
SUNDAY 12.00 RACE 1				
1 Vermeulen Chris	Ten Kate Honda	Honda CBR 1000RR	28	41'03.371
2 Chili Pierfrancesco	PSG – 1 Corse	Ducati 998 RS	28	41'07.498
3 Martin Steve	D.F.Xtreme Sterilgarda	Ducati 999 RS	28	41'09.078
4 Toseland James	Ducati Fila	Ducati 999 F04	28	41'11.718
5 Laconi Régis	Ducati Fila	Ducati 999 F04	28	41'11.761
SUNDAY 15.30 RACE 2				
1 Vermeulen Chris	Ten Kate Honda	Honda CBR 1000RR	28	40'56.568
2 Toseland James	Ducati Fila	Ducati 999 F04	28	40'57.033
3 Laconi Régis	Ducati Fila	Ducati 999 F04	28	41'10.088
4 Haga Noriyuki	Renegade Ducati	Ducati 999 RS	28	41'10.310
5 Chili Pierfrancesco	PSG – 1 Corse	Ducati 998 RS	28	41'18.338

BRANDS HATCH 01/08/2004

Brands Hatch

Name: BRANDS HATCH
Circuit length: 4197 m
Pole position: Left
Maximum slope: N.a.

Corners left: 3 Right: 6
Corner radius: min. 40°–max. 180° (approx.)
Finish line length: 380 m

Best lap	2003	Byrne Shane	Ducati 1'26.248
Superpole record	2004	Martin Steve	Ducati 1'27.213
Race record	2003	Byrne Shane	Ducati 1'26.755

Riders	Teams	Bikes	Laps	Times
SUNDAY 12.00 RACE 1				
1 Haga Noriyuki	Renegade Ducati Koji	Ducati 999 RS	25	37'08.172
2 Laconi Régis	Ducati Fila	Ducati 999 F04	25	37'08.306
3 Martin Steve	D.F.Xtreme Sterilgarda	Ducati 999 RS	25	37'10.445
4 Vermeulen Chris	Ten Kate Honda	Honda CBR 1000RR	25	37'12.923
5 Corser Troy	Foggy PETRONAS Racing	Petronas FP1	25	37'16.218
SUNDAY 12.00 RACE 1				
1 Naga Noriyuki	Renegade Ducati Koji	Ducati 999 RS	25	37'05.030
2 Chili Pierfrancesco	PSG – 1 Corse	Ducati 998 RS	25	37'05.990
3 Vermeulen Chris	Ten Kate Honda	Honda CBR 1000RR	25	37'15.669
4 Walker Chris	Foggy PETRONAS Racing	Petronas FP1	25	37'28.694
5 Ellison James	Jentin Racing	Yamaha YZF R1	25	37'29.142

ASSEN 05/09/2004

Assen

Name: TT CIRCUIT
Circuit length: 6027 m
Pole position: Left
Maximum slope: downward 0%

Corners left: 10 **Right:** 14
Corner radius: max. 175—min. 10
Finish line length: 790 m

Best lap	2003	Chili Pierfrancesco	Ducati 2'00.874
Superpole record	2003	Chili Pierfrancesco	Ducati 2'00.874
Race record	2002	Edwards Colin	Honda 2'02.395

Riders	Teams	Bikes	Laps	Times
SUNDAY 12.00 RACE 1				
1 Toseland James	Ducati Fila	Ducati 999 F04	16	33'30.741
2 Chili Pierfrancesco	PSG – 1 Corse	Ducati 998 RS	16	33'32.879
3 Laconi Régis	Ducati Fila	Ducati 999 F04	16	33'33.191
4 Haga Noriyuki	Renegade Ducati Koji	Ducati 999 RS	16	33'33.307
5 Vermeulen Chris	Ten Kate Honda	Honda CBR 1000RR	16	33'39.785
SUNDAY 12.00 RACE 2				
1 Vermeulen Chris	Ten Kate Honda	Honda CBR 1000RR	16	33'31.968
2 Toseland James	Ducati Fila	Ducati 999 F04	16	33'32.005
3 Haga Noriyuki	Renegade Ducati Koji	Ducati 999 RS	16	33'32.085
4 Chili Pierfrancesco	PSG – 1 Corse	Ducati 998 RS	16	33'35.873
5 Laconi Régis	Ducati Fila	Ducati 999 F04	16	33'38.548

IMOLA 26/09/2004

Imola

Name: IMOLA
Circuit length: 4933 m
Pole position: Left
Maximum slope: down 6.2% – up 7.81%

Corners left: 10 Right: 6
Corner radius: min. 11.60
Finish line length: 358 m

Best lap	2002	Edwards Collin	Honda 1'48.336
Superpole record	2001	Corser Troy	Aprilia 1'48.694
Race record	2002	Bayliss Troy	Ducati 1'48.389

	Riders	Teams	Bikes	Laps	Times
SUNDAY 12.00 RACE 1					
1	Laconi Régis	Ducati Fila	Ducati 999 F04	21	38'58.507
2	Vermeulen Chris	Ten Kate Honda	Honda CBR 1000RR	21	38'59.629
3	Toseland James	Ducati Fila	Ducati 999 F04	21	39'04.145
4	Naga Noriyuki	Renegade Ducati Koji	Ducati 999 RS	21	39'05.117
5	McCoy Garry	XEROX – Ducati Nortel Net.	Ducati 999 RS	21	39'10.481
SUNDAY 15.30 RACE 2					
1	Laconi Régis	Ducati Fila	Ducati 999 F04	21	39'04.926
2	Toseland James	Ducati Fila	Ducati 999 F04	21	39'04.967
3	Martin Steve	D.F.Xtreme Sterilgarda	Ducati 999 RS	21	39'17.278
4	Nannelli Gianluca	XEROX – Ducati Nortel Net.	Ducati 999 RS	21	39'28.091
5	McCoy Garry	XEROX – Ducati Nortel Net.	Ducati 999 RS	21	39'33.563

MAGNY-COURS 03/10/2004

Magny-Cours

Name: MAGNY-COURS
Circuit length: 4411 m
Pole position: Right

				Bikes	Laps	Times
Best lap		2003	Hodgson Neil	Ducati 1'40.754		
Superpole record		2003	Toseland James	Ducati 1'40.965		
Race record		2003	Hodgson Neil	Ducati 1'40.219		

	Riders	Teams	Bikes	Laps	Times
SUNDAY 12.00 RACE 1					
1	Toseland James	Ducati Fila	Ducati 999 F04	23	39'29.197
2	Haga Noriyuki	Renegade Ducati Koji	Ducati 999 RS	23	39'29.689
3	Laconi Régis	Ducati Fila	Ducati 999 F04	23	39'32.999
4	Gimbert Sebastien	Yamaha France	Yamaha YZF R1	23	39'37.024
5	Martin Steve	D.F.Xtreme Sterilgarda	Ducati 999 RS	23	39'43.023
SUNDAY 15.30 RACE 2					
1	Haga Noriyuki	Renegade Ducati Koji	Ducati 999 RS	23	39'34.329
2	Toseland James	Ducati Fila	Ducati 999 F04	23	39'37.484
3	Laconi Régis	Ducati Fila	Ducati 999 F04	23	39'40.119
4	Gimbert Sebastien	Yamaha France	Yamaha YZF R1	23	39'49.082
5	Chili Pierfrancesco	PSG – 1 Corse	Ducati 998 RS	23	39'51.836

INDEX

275